# THE
# PULSE
# TEST

**The Secret of Building Your Basic Health**

## ARTHUR F. COCA, M.D.

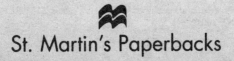

St. Martin's Paperbacks

Published by arrangement with Barricade Books Inc.

THE PULSE TEST

Library of Congress Catalog Card Number: 93-19656

ISBN: 0-312-95699-1

Printed in the United States of America

Barricade Books revised trade paperback edition published in 1994
St. Martin's Paperbacks edition/January 1996

St. Martin's Paperbacks are published by St. Martin's Press, 175 Fifth Avenue, New York, NY 10010.

10 9 8 7 6 5 4 3 2 1

I am happy to acknowledge the expert assistance that has been so generously given to the composition of this book by the late John J. O'Neill, Science Editor of the *New York Herald Tribune*.

A.C.

# Contents

# THE
# PULSE
# TEST

# Publisher's Preface

Years ago, when I was an investigative reporter, I heard that a man suffering from diabetes had put aside his insulin and was leading a normal healthy life without it.

I heard that a man who had been unsuccessfully hospitalized for an extremely painful and serious stomach ulcer was later cured of his ulcer in a matter of days. I met with him, and he was leading a happy, ulcer-free life. My curiosity was aroused when I learned that the cause of his illness had been found to be cow's milk—the very thing he had been given to "relieve" the pain. Cow's milk is a nutritious food for most people, but this man was allergic to it.

I am a skeptic by nature and training. When similar reports reached me, I sought out the physician responsible for these remarkable recoveries.

To my surprise, I discovered that what I had heard was only a small part of the whole. I was shown records of hundreds of men, women and children who had been cured of a variety of illnesses by what appeared to be a totally revolutionary approach to ill health.

I was profoundly impressed by Dr. Arthur F. Coca's astonishing results in the treatment of a long list of diseases. He appeared to have found the way to remove the cause of many illnesses rather than simply dealing with their symptoms.

I interviewed people who'd been told flatly by their doctors that "nothing can be done" to relieve one kind of affliction or another, and then, in a matter of a few weeks, they returned to good health, thanks to Dr. Coca's discoveries.

The Coca pulse-dietary method is simple but it requires dedication by patient. In the early days it was best tried under the guidance of a physician trained in the method.

As years have flown by, I have come to recognize the sad reality that American medicine is almost exclusively devoted to the treatment of symptoms. You have a headache? Your doctor will prescribe a pill to relieve it. He doesn't have time to search for what caused it.

I have also come to accept the fact that medicine is one of the most profitable businesses in America, vying only with the legal profession, dope dealing, and show business for the big incomes.

There is nothing wrong with making money, or wanting to. The tragedy is that even the most idealistic doctors—those who were drawn to medicine because they wanted to help people—find it difficult to do much in the way of preventive medicine.

To treat a patient with the pulse-test properly, a doctor would have to spend approximately three hours on the first visit and make himself available at all waking hours to answer questions.

The economics just aren't there.

I can't recall the last time I knew a doctor to make a house call, so I asked that question of my own internist.

"I think," he said, "that I made my last house call twelve years ago."

I cite all this to explain why, years ago, when I received a steady stream of queries asking "Who in my area can treat me with this method?" I was able to refer to a few doctors in the Midwest, one in the South, three in California.

One of these, a prominent physician in Missouri, wrote to me that, "I have limited respect for medical ethics. I know the value of Dr. Coca's work. My whole family has benefited from it. Yet if I dared to say publicly what I believe, I think there is a chance I would be expelled from the American Medical Association."

So, I can't refer you to a physician.

Most doctors are brainwashed. They have to believe that they know all the answers or they couldn't approach their work with such seeming confidence.

I have never met a medical doctor who knows as much about the human pulse as I do. Of course, none of them would accept this fact.

Here's one example that I found amusing. Some years ago I visited a doctor in Lakeville, Florida, to have a wart burned off each side of my waist. It was purely a vanity thing.

He did his job and then gave me an antibiotic cream.

Whatever was in that cream wasn't good for me. I developed lumps where the warts had been. I went to my friendly physician in New York and he became quite upset. He phoned a surgeon and told him he was putting me in a taxi and wanted the lumps removed "right now."

"I know Lyle, and if this isn't done today, he'll never do it!"

In the taxi I took my pulse. 74. My normal range is 60 to 78. Whatever the lumps were, they weren't upsetting my system.

The surgeon gave me a local anesthetic and operated.. He removed two lumps that very much resembled apple cores. And all the time he kept telling me that these could be malignant and I could be in big trouble.

"I'm okay," I said. I tried to explain the pulse test to him. It was like talking to a deaf man.

Before I left his office, he told me to phone him in three days for the results of the biopsy that he was ordering.

"I told you. I don't have cancer."

"Don't be a damned fool. You call me in three days."

I forgot all about it. Five days later I received an angry phone call. "You have more brass than any patient I ever treated! Why didn't you call me for the results?"

I laughed. "I know the results. I told you. I'm in excellent health. I don't have cancer."

He confirmed that fact and uttered a few expletives.

That's how much confidence I have in my pulse count as an indicator of my own health.

Unless you can find a physician remarkably different from most, you're going to have to apply the Coca technique yourself. You *can* do it yourself, safely. There are no drugs involved. You simply follow what this book tells you to do.

The method is harmless. It is also relatively simple. There are no magic elixirs and there is nothing whatsoever to purchase.

The reward for taking the pulse test and learning to heed what it tells you about yourself could mean adding ten to twenty more years to your life. And I'm talking about years free of high blood pressure, heart attacks, headaches and a score of other ailments.

This is the only book Dr. Coca ever wrote for laymen. Much of what is in this book appeared in technical language in a scientific medical work of which three editions were published half-a-century ago.

Dr. Coca was not your ordinary hand-holding physician. He was pure scientist. He had no bedside manner and no patience with foolishness.

As an author myself, I knew that forty to sixty thousand books a year are published—and that most are consigned to oblivion even as they are trucked from the binderies. After working with Dr. Coca on this manuscript, I found three publishers eager to publish.

One offered a $2,000 advance, which in those days wasn't bad.

The reason I found publishers so willing was that at the time I was business manager of a group of comic magazines for my dear friend, the late Bill Gaines. I had helped turn a ten-cent comic book into a quarter magazine—and *Mad* went on to make millions upon millions of dollars. So book publishers, no less supersti-

tious than other people, now perceived me as a man with
a Midas touch.

At about this point in my life I won a libel suit against
Walter Winchell. After legal costs I was left with $21,500.
That was more money than I ever had before.

I spoke to the publisher most interested in publishing
*The Pulse Test.* I listened to his plan to promote the book.
He really didn't have one. He would take a small ad in the
Sunday book section of *The New York Times* costing about
$600. If nothing happened, it would probably be "good-
bye Pulse Test."

I believed in Dr. Coca and his discoveries. I felt they
were too important to be lost. So I took $8,000 of my
libel winnings and published *The Pulse Test* myself. I had
never published a book before. I had zero knowledge of
book publishing.

My first hurdle was to persuade the censorship (they
call it "acceptability") department of *The New York Times*
to allow me to run an ad for the book. I was referred to
their house physician.

He phoned the New York Academy of Medicine. He
wanted them to give him an excuse not to accept the ad.
The method was quackery. It was untested. It was
unsound. Anything.

He was somewhat frustrated. "We have no comment,"
he was told.

"Do you agree we shouldn't run this ad?"

"No comment," he was told again.

He phoned the national office of the American Medical
Association. He received that same stonewalling.

"Son of a gun," he said. "You go ahead and run the ad."

Why was there no comment? Well, it would take many pages to list Dr. Coca's professional accomplishments. Suffice it to say that for seventeen years he was medical director of Lederle Laboratories, one of the largest pharmaceutical houses in the world. He was Honorary President of the American Association of Immunologists. He was founder and first editor of the *Journal of Immunology* which is the foremost medical publication in its field.

He taught at Cornell, the University of Pennsylvania and Post-Graduate studies at Columbia University.

He was a member of the American Society for the Study of Allergy; the Society for Experimental Biology and Medicine; the Society of American Bacteriologists; the American Association for Cancer Research; the Harvey Society; the New Jersey Medical Society; the Society for the Study of Asthma and Allied Conditions; the William Pepper Medical Society, and Alpha Omega Alpha.

He contributed to *Tice's Practice of Medicine* and wrote extensively for medical journals throughout the world. Among the editorial boards on which he served were those of the *Journal of Allergy,* the *Journal of Investigative Dermatology,* and the *Journal of Applied Nutrition.*

The medical societies didn't dare say a negative word about him.

The ad, written by one of today's giants in the advertising agency business, pulled poorly.

I don't give up easily. I sat down and wrote my own ad.

To date *The Pulse Test* has sold more than 125,000 copies. It has been published in Germany, France, Japan and England. But this book launched a publishing house that I would sell many years later for $12,000,000.

When *The Pulse Test* was originally published in 1956,

I didn't want to become a book publisher and hadn't planned on it.

In 1957, I published two books. In 1958, I published three books.

Since that time the Lyle Stuart imprint has appeared on millions of books that have changed the lives and attitudes of many people.

These have included the works of Dr. Albert Ellis, whose *Sex Without Guilt* launched the worldwide sexual revolution; *The Sensuous Woman* which sold more than 600,000 copies in cloth and more than 10,000,000 in paperback in the United States alone; *The Rich and the Super-Rich* by Ferdinand Lundberg, which told a whole generation who really owns America; *The Great Quotations* compiled by that crusading journalist George Seldes; *The Washington Pay-Off,* which exposed the payola of Senators and Congressmen. Although names were named and specific bribes cited, the whole thing seemed too hard to believe. (It pre-dated Watergate and Abscam.) *Where Did I Come From?* is the most popular book ever published on sex education for children.

These are a few of the more than twenty-five hundred titles I have published in thirty years.

Yet, when asked, "What is the most important book you've ever published?" I unhesitatingly reply, "*The Pulse Test* by Dr. Arthur Coca."

I believe this more strongly than I can convey in words. Here is no blind faith doctrine. Here is an approach that can be tested and proven again and again.

I recall being part of a standing-room-only crowd at the New School for Social Research which was attended by delegates from fourteen nations.

"Do you believe this method will ever be widely adopted?" one of them asked.

"I wish I could tell you that I do," Dr. Coca replied. "I'm a realist. As long as the profit is in the treatment of symptoms rather than in the search for causes, that's where the medical profession will go for its harvest."

Let me tell you two anecdotes.

In 1928 Dr. Coca and his wife established the first blood bank in America. Its laboratory was in Manhattan. Finally, things reached the point where there were no funds to continue.

Dr. Coca wrote a letter, which was published in *The New York Times*, mourning the fact that in this great nation, there were not the means to continue something so important.

On the morning that the letter appeared in the *Times*, a man climbed the two flights of stairs that led to offices of the Blood Transfusion Association of New York.

"Dr. Coca, I read your letter. How much does it cost to keep your blood bank going?"

Coca cited the monthly cost.

The man took out his checkbook. "Dr. Coca, my name is John D. Rockefeller. Here is a check to keep you going for another year."

Dr. Coca managed to keep it going for eleven years.

You couldn't ever say anything bad about the Rockefellers to Arthur or Ella Coca!

The second story is more meaningful and doesn't have as happy an ending.

In the days before passenger planes, Dr. Coca would convene an annual meeting of the top allergists in

America. They would arrive by train and automobile from all over the country. They'd meet at Dr. Coca's home to exchange their latest findings.

Dr. Coca, a true pioneer, knew the importance of sharing knowledge.

One year, a dozen or so top medical men sat on his enclosed porch in Oradell, New Jersey.

"I have something to tell you," Dr. Coca began. "I believe I have made a very important discovery."

He went on to talk about what he had found about the human pulse. He described several of the half a hundred cases he'd treated successfully.

Dr. Coca told me, "When I was finished, they were all silent. I invited them into my living room to see the research and the case histories.

"Nobody moved. Not one man stood up to follow me. Looking back, I guess they thought I was crazy. That moment gave me the biggest shock in my life."

"I never called another annual meeting. Years later when the Society which I had founded celebrated its quarter-century anniversary, I was invited to be the guest of honor. I wrote a letter declining and said, "If some of the men sitting on the porch that night had followed me into my living room, they might well be alive today and able to attend your dinner!"

Although, the Mayo brothers indicated to Arthur Coca that he was in poor health at the age of 62, with not much longer to live, he went on to enjoy excellent health to the age of 84, thanks to his pulse test.

He lives on in these pages. When I tried to let *The Pulse Test* go "out of print" I found that I couldn't. Word of mouth recommendations from people whose lives had been helped sent others in search of copies.

A monumental discovery had been made.

This book is an attempt to spread the good word.

In the pages that follow, Dr. Coca opens the door to the prevention and cure of a host of illnesses. You have but to enter.

LYLE STUART

*New York City*
*August, 1993*

A Postscript: Much has been accomplished by medicine and scientific technology since this book was originally written and published.

It would be tempting and relatively easy to revise sections to incorporate up-to-the-minute medical approaches. However, after careful consideration, I've overcome this temptation for the following reason.

*The Pulse Test* is a classic. To revise or update it would be to deprive the reader of the rich value that this book contained more than forty years ago when it was first written for publication—and which it contains today. The reader is entitled to that—and so I've left the contents virtually unchanged.

# Foreword:

## What Allergy Really Is

An editorial in a medical journal said that he who would define allergy must write a book. You have a book in your hands, but we will not waste pages on definitions.

Rather let's concentrate on your health.

You will find in these pages that allergy means something far more important to your health and to the length of your life than you ever possibly imagined.

Before you are done with this book, you will know that allergy no longer means merely hay-fever or asthma or an outbreak of hives. It can also mean high blood pressure, diabetes, epileptic seizures and stammering. It means "that tired feeling, constipation, stomach ulcer, spells of dizziness, headaches and mental depression. In truth, it may mean much of what ails the health and happiness of human beings.

However, the book would fail of its chief purpose if it merely explained allergy. Much more important, it tells you what to do about it.

The visiting doctor can hardly leave his patient without

having used his thermometer, his stethoscope and his watch.

With his watch he times the pulse. But as often as he does this in his busy career it is exceptional for him to use the pulse count either to diagnose the illness or to plan its relief.

The pulse has been almost totally neglected as an indicator of ill health. Yet this simplest of all the methods of examination is the key to some of the deepest mysteries of man's existence—the key with which he may emancipate himself from ill health.

If you can count to 100 and are determined to be well, you can go a long way toward eliminating your allergic troubles if you are a usual case. By "usual case" I mean chiefly the so-called neurotic people who suffer constantly recurring or persistent headache, "indigestion," constipation, tiredness, occasional dizziness, stuffy nose, who have consulted one or more physicians, among them perhaps a "specialist," and have been told that their health is excellent, but that they are "nervous," and since they are incurable they should help themselves by keeping their minds off their symptoms—"forget them." Such persons can almost always be permanently relieved of their miseries through the pulse-dietary tests described in this book.

In the deliverance of the "neurotic" person, then, the first step to be learned is counting the pulse; and this is very easy to do. Many young children learn in one-minute demonstrations at school or in first-aid courses how to find the pulse. It is the rare adult who has not found his pulse merely by copying the doctor. The following detailed instructions for finding the pulse will therefore be unnecessary for most readers.

The pulse can be felt at many spots on the body, and the rate, at any given moment, is the same in all of them.

The most convenient spot is at the wrist an inch and a half above the base of the thumb. Place the left hand (if you are right-handed) in the lap with the palm facing up. Then place the first two fingers of the right hand on the wrist so that their average distance is about an inch an a half from the base of the thumb, and three quarters of an inch from the end of the wrist.

Some veins may be seen under the surface of the skin, but these are not what you want to feel as there is just a steady flow of blood in them and no pulse-beat. The pulse-beat is felt in the arteries, and there is an artery in the wrist at a lower depth than that of the visible veins. It carries the blood coming directly from the heart, and as the heart forces the blood through the body with strokes like a force-pump, you can feel the pump-pulses of the heart in the arteries.

The artery in the wrist lies between the sinews in the middle of the upper surface of the wrist and the bone at the outer side of the wrist. Only a slight pressure on the finger-tips is usually required in order to feel the pulse. Move the fingers around slightly and vary the pressure a little until the pulse is detected.

Once the pulse is found there will be no further difficulty in locating the right spot.

When counting your pulse have a watch or clock with a second hand close in view. Pick up the pulse with the finger-tips and wait until the second hand reaches 60.

Then count 1 on the next pulse-beat and continue counting the beats until the second hand has made a complete circuit and returned to 60, which will mark the completion of the minute. The number of the pulse-beats counted in one minute is the pulse-rate.

In the quarter of a century since this book was originally written, modern technology has produced a variety of gadgets now on the market that show your pulse beat in an instant. Most are reasonably priced and will make pulse-counting easier.

It will be necessary to count your pulse many times in the course of the test, but this task is not at all difficult, and the beneficial results which will follow the close adherence to the test-diet and pulse schedule will be more than an adequate return for your effort.

What you are buying is not merely relief from present ailment, but, if you are successful, also health insurance and life extension.

The diagnostic method outlined in this volume is fundamentally simple. It is based on the fact that allergens speed up the pulse. It consists essentially of testing isolated foods *in order to tell which ones accelerate the pulse.*

On the day the test is started, each "meal" may be limited to a single, simple food. (You may have many "meals" throughout the day.) The pulse is counted in the morning before rising and again just before the first meal. Thirty minutes after the meal the pulse is counted, and again at sixty minutes after the meal.

Immediately after the 60 minute count another single food is eaten and again the pulse-count is taken after the two half-hour intervals; and so on through the day.

A record is kept of the foods eaten and of the pulse-counts. The injurious foods are recognized by the abnormal speed-up of the pulse. When these foods are dropped from the diet the allergic symptoms often disappear as if by magic.

That in essence is the procedure.

Later I will describe the "normal" pulse. The following preliminary facts are helpful to anyone making a first attempt to interpret a pulse-dietary record.

A number of competent medical scientists in this country and abroad (London, Zurich, Madrid), after applying this method of examination in hundreds of cases of many common ailments, are agreed concerning the following features of the *normal* pulse-rate:

1. The pulse-rate in the normal person is not affected at all by digestion, nor by *ordinary* physical activity, nor by normal emotional influences. It is remarkably stable.

2. If a person is not suffering sunburn or an infection such as common cold, any variation from his normal pulse-rate in usual activity is probably due to an allergic reaction.

The pulse, then, may be considered a dependable first watchdog of our health-citadel. It tells us promptly whenever we are in possibly injurious contact with our allergic enemies.

# (1)

## First Steps...

It is my main purpose to describe to you a novel concept of the causes of a number of the most important diseases of mankind, including migraine headaches, high blood pressure, diabetes and heart attacks.

This new concept is nothing less than a reasonable and easily understood explanation of the single common *cause* of all of these symptoms.

This same single cause is responsible for a number of other relatively minor symptoms—indigestion, heartburn, hives, neuralgia, abnormal tiredness, spells of dizziness, constipation, nasal stuffiness and probably many others—which constitute so large a part of the human physical afflictions.

Having learned what provokes these illnesses, we can completely overcome them in most cases by mere avoidance of their causes.

I shall attempt with a minimum of technical language to show that it is not at all difficult for lay people of average intelligence, from the age of ten or twelve years upward, to understand this procedure, and to take decisive responsibility for its technical application in their own persons under the direction of a skilled diagnostician. *Indeed, the new technic usually cannot be successful without the patient's faithful cooperation, and his understanding of every step of the investigation.*

I want to present now a bare outline of the history and the fundamentals of this new method of medical diagnosis.

Many years ago, my wife, who was actively engaged in medical research, and in the direction of an important medical service, was suddenly stricken with an attack of angina pectoris. This incapacitated her for three years. Two heart specialists gloomily predicted the end of her life within five years.

The immediate cause of the attack was a dose of a morphine derivative which usually quiets the pulse, but which in this instance caused it to speed up to three times the normal rate—the nurse reporting, "A pulse of 180—couldn't count beyond that—it just flowed."

When, on my next visit to Mrs. Coca, I looked at her bed chart, I said: "That was quite a jump your pulse took."

Mrs. Coca agreed. And then she added thoughtfully, "Now that you mention it, my heart races after some meals."

"That's interesting," I remarked. "Why don't we check your pulse following single foods?"

Mrs. Coca replied, "Why not?"

An examination of a pulse record taken in this manner showed *initially* that only three foods send her pulse above 68. (Potato sent her pulse above 180.)

Soon after this first attack there were others, and she noticed that the worst occurred within a short time (minutes) after the eating of certain foods (beef, potato). We then observed that after eating these foods she always showed a decided acceleration of the pulse, and I used this means of judging which foods were injurious and which were safe.

If ever urgent necessity has mothered an invention, this was such an occasion. After a long, often discouraging search the following small list of tolerated foods was found: Fowl, fish, peas, string beans, chocolate, milk, cheese, wheat, rye, rice, tea, coffee, figs, grapes, honey, cane sugar, yeast; just about enough to make her able— and willing—to live.

She became free from heart-pain so long as she observed the dietary restrictions, and she performed ordinary housework and gardening without becoming over-tired. More important, she resumed her indispensable collaboration in my medical research.

We could have been satisfied with this happy outcome of the experiment, but, fortunately as it certainly was for the development of the new idea, my wife had suffered many years from a number of other afflictions which she had accepted as part of her genetic inheritance. These were migraine, colitis, attacks of dizziness and fainting, abnormal tiredness and indigestion.

As time passed after her many food-allergens were recognized and eliminated from her diet, she realized that all of those miseries also were gone. She did not tell me this until she was sure, and when she did I recognized at once the possible scope of application of the new method of investigation.

Van Leewenhoek, centuries ago, could not have been more deeply thrilled—and awed—at his first view of the strange new world of the microorganisms through his famous microscope than I was at this vision of the new medicine, which leaped to my mind with my wife's assured statement.

Recognizing then the allergic nature of all her symptoms, I quickly began to apply the accidentally acquired knowledge to the relief of migraine and indigestion in other persons.

Soon I was obliged to include many other symptoms in the category of allergy, since, after the "treatment," these disappeared with those already identified as allergic.

Here is the list of the symptoms which I have successfully treated as allergic:

| | |
|---|---|
| recurrent headache | abnormal tiredness |
| nervousness | indigestion |
| migraine | (vomiting, gas, nausea) |
| dizziness | neuralgia |
| constipation | sinusitis |
| canker sores | hypertension |
| heartburn | hives |
| epilepsy | heart attacks (angina) |
| overweight | asthma |
| underweight | hemorrhoids |
| irritability | psychic depression |
| gastric ulcer | diabetes |
| abdominal pain | chest pain |
| gallbladder pain | gastro-intestinal bleeding |
| gastric pain | conjunctivitis |
| nervous and emotional | nose bleed |
| instability (neurasthenia) | colitis |

Keep in mind that the allergic nature of these manifestations was not proved by the mere fact that they all disappeared after certain foods were kept from the diet, although this happy result undoubtedly stands as strongly supporting evidence. In most instances there were also three other kinds of corroborative evidence.

Firstly, many of the sufferers exhibited more than one of the above-mentioned conditions, and in most cases all of the existing symptoms disappeared.

Secondly, in most instances the symptoms could be brought on at will by merely restoring the offending foods to the diet.

Thirdly, *without exception*, the symptoms were accompanied by a speeding up of the heart-beat.

### Representative Cases

Let us review some of these remarkable recoveries which will illustrate what I have been saying.

Mr. G. is the proprietor of an automobile-repair shop, who was suffering from severe three-day attacks of migraine at about two-week intervals. During the attacks he was confined to bed, wholly incapacitated. There was also indigestion, heartburn, swelling of the face, and a physical tiredness that was almost constantly present.

It was soon found that his chief food-allergens were wheat, cane-sugar and coffee. Strangely, wheat and cane-sugar caused headache without swelling of the face, whereas coffee did not cause headache but did cause swelling of the face and lips. All of these three foods caused an accelerated heartbeat. This man's attacks of migraine and the other symptoms stopped as soon as the three foods were dropped from his diet, and in the succeeding many years he has experienced mild symptoms only when he deliberately ate one of those foods.

Mrs. B., a wealthy widow of 70-odd years, was almost bedridden by marked physical tiredness and migratory neuralgia. She had been troubled for "over 30 years" with overweight and constipation, and each winter suffered protracted colds.

She had withdrawn from social activity, and was in a state of psychic depression. In the pulse-dietary examination, which lasted for three weeks, the following food-allergens were identified: Milk, orange, melon, peanut, lemon, carrot, beet, asparagus and onion. These foods were eliminated from her diet, and immediately all the symptoms disappeared. She has not suffered an attack of cold, and has lost 35 lbs. of her overweight since that time. She resumed her social life and became the active chairwoman of her local Red Cross unit.

B. B. is a young man who had withdrawn from college on account of frequently recurring epileptic seizures. A well-known drug, even in doses of five capsules daily, did not prevent daily minor seizures and frequent major ones. His mind had become "foggy." The following foods were found to cause an increased heart-beat; cereals (especially wheat), orange, pineapple and asparagus. Seizures ceased completely as soon as these foods were avoided, and he was able to obtain employment. The drug was discontinued.

One evening, three months after he had begun to practice that avoidance, he deliberately ate a quantity of bread. On arising the next morning he suffered a major seizure. In the next six months there was no attack until he again ate wheat (spaghetti) one evening. On arising the next morning he experienced a major seizure, breaking a tooth.

Only then did he become convinced of the direct relationship of his food-allergy to the epileptic seizures, and of his ability to prevent them. With this knowledge he decided to return to college, and he has since graduated. Other allergic symptoms in this patient were headache, abnormal tiredness, neuralgia and nervousness. All of these ceased after elimination of his food-allergens.

The technic of the new method of diagnosis is fairly simple, and it can usually be applied without interruption of your daily occupation.

The interpretation of the pulse-record in the first few days of serial tests consists in a succession of tentative guesses to be confirmed or changed as the tests continue.

The first guess concerns the normal low count, and in this you may be very far from the truth. Rarely the lowest observed count in the allergic period is below the actual normal, as determined after all of the allergens have been eliminated. More often the normal low is never reached in the early days of the tests.

Nevertheless this guess, even if wrong at first, must be made because the decisions concerning the test must be made with reference to that basic figure.

Usually the major food allergens reveal themselves in the unmistakable speeding-up of the pulse shortly after they are eaten; and as these are eliminated from the diet the general level of the pulse tends to drop, and with it the lowest count.

The drastic changes in one's estimate of the normal pulse-range that must sometimes be made can be discomforting to the diagnostician, and startling to the allergic patient. Initial ranges of 66 to 102, 74 to 116 and 76 to 106 have been seen to drop to normal ranges of 54 to 66, 60 to 72, and 58 to 76 respectively.

The outcome of the tests has been occasionally disconcerting. I could hardly credit my ears when one of the early migraine-sufferers reported a pulse rate of only 45. Since then I have seen three other instances of rates below 50. On the other hand there have been a number of records showing normal rates up to 80 or more, *but not higher than 84,* which is the allergy deadline. Any count above 84, in children or adults, if taken when the patient is quiet and has no infection such as a cold, has usually been a sign of allergy.

In two instances of strongly suspected allergy the test showed a normal range of the pulse-rate for several days. In both cases my confidence in the test wavered temporarily. However, I learned that in both individuals there were no symptoms during that period for the simple reason that by chance they had missed eating any of their few food allergens.

The younger one had suffered from distressing attacks of hives. These had ceased after the test was started and after the first day he had chosen his own diet. For five days his pulse remained level. At last he suffered an outbreak of hives, which he mistakenly attributed to orange. Believing that he had identified the cause of his trouble he discontinued the tests. He completely ignored his occasional abdominal discomforts which he had not mentioned, and which then recurred, and a few weeks later became acute, resembling appendicitis.

Surgery revealed that the trouble was not an infected appendix, but an inflamed large bowel, a condition which was recognized by the surgeon and the attending physician as being allergic in nature. The tests were resumed and his single food-allergen, ginger, was finally detected. He was fond of ginger ale; also in the two days just previous to the attack he had indulged in pumpkin pie richly spiced with ginger.

The young man now understands the importance of completing the food-tests. He also appreciates the hereditary significance of his allergy, since his father suffered from gastric ulcer, gastritis and hemorrhoids, all of which were proved to be allergic in origin, and were cured with the same tests.

Most disturbing is the patient whose pulse remains in the high allergic range, no matter what he eats. Unfornately this result may have divergent causes; either the individual is allergic to all or nearly all foods that he has tested, or he is not affected by any food but by one or more air-carried dusts or vapors to which he is continually exposed. In the former case the difficulty can usually be resolved with the aid of a minor nerve-cutting operation (sympathectomy), which simply abolishes many of the food-sensitivities. In the latter, the problem of locating the elusive offender is sometimes heartbreaking and may be practically insoluble.

There is one still mysterious phenomenon of food allergy that confuses the allergic sufferer until he gets acquainted with it and learns how to use it. For example,

Mrs. A. S. experienced symptoms and a fast pulse from her test with peas and beans which she was in the habit of eating frequently. After two weeks she retested peas, and on the next day she reported a completely negative reaction; no pains, pulse quiet.

Since the results of the first test had been unequivocal she was told that the sensitivity to pea had probably disappeared in the intervening two weeks, and that the present test would probably revive it; this could be proved by a pea test on the following day.

Intrigued by the experimental problem Mrs. A. S. carried out the test and was actually pleased over the rather painful confirmation of the prediction. She is allergic to fifteen foods, five of which, including cane sugar, she is unable to eat at all. (She is not allergic to beet sugar.) However, through methodical experiment she has found that the other ten can be eaten at about one week intervals with impunity. In the five years since the survey, her health has been perfect.

The stories that I have just told you are not "fairy-tales." They illustrate the sober truth that, by scientific approach, there has been discovered an almost mathematically accurate means of determining the cause of a long list of the most dreadful afflictions of the human flesh; and of course, the means of ending these miseries by meticulous avoidance of their identified causes.

Two objections have been raised against the practice of the patient counting his own pulse. One of these is that the layman is not capable of taking an accurate pulse-count, but this is completely refuted by the practical results of the procedure in hundreds of cases. It is easier to teach an intelligent child twelve years old or even younger to count the pulse satisfactorily than it is to teach a diabetic person to administer insulin to himself as many are obliged to do.

Also, as mentioned earlier, there are several gadgets on the market that will show you your pulse rate in seconds.

The second criticism warns that counting one's pulse tends to aggravate a neurotic state, or even bring it on. It is thought unwise to encourage the sick to think about their health. This is true when the cause of their ailment is unknown. However, when the victim of hypertension or migraine-headache or dizziness learns that these conditions are curable, and that the cure lies at his fingertips, his fears vanish, and he finds himself confronted by a fascinating problem, the solution of which will almost certainly turn out to be unique—his personal answer. He learns that the procedure is a game with high stakes, present and future, in which the player has a wonderful chance of winning. It is nearly always the quitter who loses.

Many of you know that in some allergic conditions, especially hay-fever, the particular exciting cause or causes—that is, the pollens—can be identified through tests in the skin with properly prepared pollen-extracts. You may be wondering why I have not availed myself of this mode of examination. The answer to this query is that the skin-test has often been tried in many of the conditions that we are considering, but with regularly unsatisfactory results.

Curiously this failure of the skin to react in conditions that are under the strongest suspicion of being allergic in nature has had an opposite influence upon two groups of physicians. To the allergists the negative skin-test means that the condition is not allergic. To many internists, other medical specialists and general practitioners such a negative reaction in obviously allergic patients discredits the concept, or at least the practice of allergy.

Some allergists have hoped vaguely for some kind of test that would extend the diagnostic function to cover symptoms which they suspect to be allergic in certain instances. However, the results of the pulse test that I have just described have necessitated so great an extension of the concept of allergic disease that only a few specialists have ventured to accept the test as the answer to their hope.

# (2)

# The Allergy Mystery Solved

Allergies have their mysteries, but medical science has solved many of them, saving countless patients from lives of misery, and restoring many of them to a comfortable existence, if not always to full robust health.

Four armies of allergies are known to have been waging war on human beings. We now discover that there is a fifth column of allergies, more numerous and more dangerous than the others, whose very existence was unknown to us. These underground makers of ills and ailments have now been exposed, not as part and parcel of our normal individual make-up, citizens, so to speak, of our physical economy, but as unnecessary aliens to whom we have given passports that we can revoke.

Now that we know them we can deal with them.

The method is simple. If you are lucky you may learn the principal cause or causes of your ailments in a week or two. Sometimes longer time is required, and one in twenty persons needs a relatively minor nerve-operation, which abolishes most of their food-sensitivities entirely.

Let us now examine the four kinds of allergic diseases that have been mentioned.

1. The first of these is commonly known as the hay-fever group. Also in this group are asthma and eczema. The disease is hereditary, and only descendants of the "hay-fever family" are affected by any of these three conditions.

The familiar skin-tests used by allergists to detect the presence of allergic antibodies apply only to this group.

The hereditary factor which controls and unites this group affects about one-tenth of the people.

2. The second kind of allergic disease is known as contact-dermatitis; and it is most commonly caused by poison-ivy and related plants. It can be caused also by primrose, some pollens, various vegetable oils such as the oil of orange and turpentine, and by some chemicals.

Allergic antibodies are not present in the blood.

The skin is the only body-tissue that is affected by this form of allergy; this poison-ivy leaf can be swallowed (in small quantity) with impunity by the allergic person provided the leaf does not touch the lips or skin.

About 70 percent of all human beings are susceptible to poison-ivy.

3. The third kind is the allergy-of-infection, which is typified by tuberculin-sensitivity. Since everyone who has been visited by the tubercule bacillus sustains some degree of infection (though most of us recover), the vast majority of us become tuberculin sensitive, and so we exhibit a "positive" reaction to the tuberculin test.

This sensitivity does no harm. However, the infectious allergy which many of us acquire toward those fungi that cause "athlete's foot" is directly injurious because it is only through the allergy that the fungi, growing in the outer layer of the skin, are able to harm us.

4. Serum sickness (skin-eruption, fever, joint-pains, etc.) sometimes follows injection of antitoxin.

The greater part of all people are susceptible.

The greater part of this book concerns itself not with any of these four recognized kinds of allergic disease, but with the fifth group which has recently been identified, and to which I have given the specific designation "idioblapsis," a word derived from the two Greek roots; "idio," meaning an individual quality, and "blapsis," meaning spoiler. Thus, "a spoiler peculiar to the individual."

This group is by far the most important to men and women. It is the one that you and I should be most interested in because it affects more than 90 percent of the population of the United States. It is distinguished from the other four by the following features:

a. Allergic antibodies cannot be detected. Thus, skin tests are negative, and are not useful in discovering the harmful foods.

b. It is controlled by an hereditary character that seems to be distinct from that of the hay-fever group.

c. Its symptoms are characteristic.

d. Contact with the causes is regularly followed by the quickening of the pulse-rate.

This fifth group was originally called "food-allergy," which emphasizes the food-allergens as its most common and important excitants or causes. However, I had better mention some of the non-dietary allergens of this group which may be important, and sometimes even the sole excitants of severe allergic symptoms in some individuals.

Among those most commonly found guilty is tobacco. In some people tobacco causes indigestion and diarrhea, abnormal tiredness and painful menstruation and many other symptoms. A large part of the population are allergic to the fabric-dust ("house-dust") in rugs, mattresses, upholstery, etc. Some persons have been found allergic to lipstick, perfumes, mentholated nose-drops, headache medicines, laxatives, soap-powder, coal-gas, fumes of paint and cement, and wood-smoke. In one case (a physician's mother) the cause of her constipation that was finally detected was her laxative containing cascara. As soon as she stopped taking the laxative she became and remained regular.

The harassed victims of food-allergy are painfully, or at least disagreeably aware of the fact that practically every part of the body is vulnerable to "food-allergy," and they never cease to marvel, however disgustedly, at the variety of the avenues through which their allergens may gain access to distant susceptible parts of the body.

Consider, for example, the case of the woman who could not be exposed to the exhaust-fumes of a bus without suffering urgent colicky diarrhea; the young woman who suffered abnormal tiredness and sinusitis from the use of a *certain* lipstick; the two epileptic girls who suffered mild seizures after inhaling tobacco smoke (not of their own making); the woman who suffered an asthmatic attack within a matter of minutes after the application to her forehead of a solution of a drug to which she was allergic; and the physician who suffered migraine and an accelerated pulse soon after the injection into his skin of extremely minute amounts of milk, egg, and orange, to all of which he is very allergic, although the skin itself showed no reaction. There is also the young woman incapacitated on account of painful swelling of feet and legs due only to chewing a gum containing aspirin.

All of the five groups of allergic disease, as well as a similar experimental condition known as anaphylaxis are found in lower animals.

Dr. Fred W. Wittich in Minneapolis beautifully documented the occurrence of hay-fever (ragweed) in dogs. My former colleague, Dr. Charles R. Schroeder, described allergic eczema, rhinitis, etc., due to cow's milk, in a young walrus. The British allergist Dr. Bray reported hay-fever in cattle. Allergy of infection (ringworm) is common in lower animals; and Landsteiner, with Merrill Chase, described experimental ivy dermatitis in guinea-pigs, the late Henry W. Straus making a similar report of experiments in monkeys. Serum-sickness was long ago observed in cattle and in horses, and more recently by Moyer Fleischer of St. Louis, in rabbits.

We see then that our allergic disease is not a special punishment visited by Nature upon erring mankind; it is merely another mark of our humble origin.

And only now are we beginning to understand it.

# (3)

# The Pulse Test

The pulse-dietary system has become a special medical diagnostic art. It is based on a simple, easily-proven premise; that your pulse-rate is often accelerated by foods and other substances; that the reason the pulse is accelerated is because your system is allergic to that which is making your pulse race; and that life-spoiling and life-shortening conditions such as migraine, eczema, epilepsy, diabetes, and hypertension may be caused by your continuing to expose yourself to those foods or substances to which you are allergic.

A very small number of doctors have investigated this premise. Many of these have adopted its methods of preventive treatment; some of them in foreign countries.

When you telephone for your first appointment with a doctor who practices this technique, you should be given the following instructions:

1. You *must* stop smoking entirely until the cigarette test, which will be made later.

2. You count your pulse (one minute) a) just before each meal; b) three times after each meal at half-hour intervals; c) just before retiring; d) just after waking, before rising in the morning. All pulse counts are to be made sitting except the important one on waking. This is made before you sit up.

3. You record all the items you eat at each meal.

4. You continue the pulse-dietary records for two or three days with the usual three meals.

5. You then make *single-food* tests for two or more whole days in this way; beginning early in the morning after the "before rising" count, and continuing for 12 to 14 hours, you eat a *small* portion of a different single food *every hour*. For example, slice of bread, glass of milk, orange, 2 tablespoonfuls of sugar in water, a few dried prunes (or a peach), egg, potato, coffee, meat, apple, banana, carrot (raw), celery, cabbage (raw), onion, coffee (black), date, cucumber, nuts, other meats (plain), chocolate (sweet), grape (or raisin), corn (frozen), etc. You count the pulse just before each eating, and again one half hour later. Do not test any food that is known to disagree.

6. You bring the whole record with you for your first appointment, which may last two or three hours, and which is not spent in examinations (those having been made by other competent clinical diagnosticians), but in explanations of the pulse-dietary method.

A physician who is experienced in the interpretation of the pulse-dietary record can usually determine from the examination of your records, at the time of the appointment, whether the solution of your case will be relatively easy or difficult. A few easy cases have been entirely solved at this single appointment; the resulting instructions brought complete and lasting freedom from all the allergic symptoms.

After she had read the first edition of this book, a New Hampshire woman wrote to me to express her gratitude. She had long suffered severe morning migraines. Both of the physicians in her small town had examined and treated her; both suggested she see a psychiatrist.

"I knew it wasn't mental and I knew I wasn't crazy," she wrote. "I came upon your book and immediately applied myself. I determined my normal pulse range. On waking, my range was normal. But a short time later my pulse had jumped from 78 to 104 and before I had put anything in my mouth, the headaches began.

"For three days in a row this occurred. I couldn't believe it. What was I missing? What was I overlooking?

"I decided to note every move I made. I woke with a pad and pencil next to my bed. I wrote the following: 'Awakened. Took pulse. Sat up and took pulse. Put robe and slippers on. Walked to bathroom. Used toilet. Washed face and hands. Brushed teeth—' and suddenly a chill went through me. I *was* putting something into my mouth. Toothpaste. The same brand of toothpaste I'd used for years.

"The next morning I switched to another brand of toothpaste. That was several weeks ago and I haven't had another migraine headache in all that time!"

Unusual? Yes. This woman may be the only person in the world allergic to that brand of toothpaste. But allergic she was and she paid a painful price for it.

### Technic of the Pulse-Test

Each human individual differs from all others in his entirety and in at least most of his component characters, such as the "finger prints." It should not be surprising then to learn that the "pulse-character" is also individually different—often widely so.

The individual *normal* pulse-character can be practically defined by the pulse-rate (beats per minute) in two or perhaps three respects. 1) the average level; 2) the range (or "pulse-differential," Sanchez-Cuenca), that is the difference between the daily low rate and high rate; and 3) the slight variations in the daily maximal rate (not greater than two beats per minute).

### Examples

|                    | Individual A | Individual B | Individual C |
|--------------------|:------------:|:------------:|:------------:|
| Low rate           | 40           | 60           | 68           |
| Maximum            | 52           | 52           | 82 — 84      |
| Pulse-differential | 12           | 2            | 14 — 16      |

No normal maximum above 84 has been observed.

The pulse may be counted wherever it can be felt—usually at the wrist, but also in the neck, at the temple, etc. In some hospitals it is customary to count the beat through 15 seconds and multiply that number by four. For the "pulse-test" that estimate is *not* sufficiently accurate, since a difference of only one or two beats in the whole minute count is frequently significant for the diagnosis. Hence, the allergic person has been advised to count the pulse for a whole minute; and a glance at the record tells the examiner whether that instruction has been followed. For whole-minute counts frequently show odd numbers; half-minute counts multiplied by 2, of course, never.

The first object of the tests is to determine the individual's normal low pulse-rate, and one would think that that rate should be observed on waking after a night's rest, as is often the case. However, that would not be the case if the individual happens to be allergic to the "dust" in his bedding, especially mattress or pillow; or if a powerful food-allergen, eaten before retiring or at dinner continues to affect the pulse through the night—a frequent occurrence.

From the beginning of the testing, then, the individual notes the lowest counts as they occur, and changes his estimate of the normal low as the count descends.

A second object of the test is to determine the individual's normal maximum pulse-rate, at least approximately. This can be done only on the basis of the record of counts made at least 14 times through 12 hours (at least) each day.

*Examples*

| A.M. DAY | allergic to tobacco only | | | | | | Mrs. K. menstrual period | | | | | | |
|---|---|---|---|---|---|---|---|---|---|---|---|---|---|
| | 0 | 1 | 2 | 3 | 4 | 5 | 6 | 0 | 1 | 2 | 4 | 6 | 8 | 10 |
| BR | | 68 | 60 | 60 | 60 | 60 | 60 | | 64 | 60 | 64 | 60 | 60 | 60 |
| BKFST. | | 84 | 72 | 68 | 68 | 68 | 64 | | 62 | 58 | 60 | 64 | 62 | 64 |
| 30 min. | | 88 | 72 | 76 | 72 | 68 | 68 | | 60 | 80 | 64 | 64 | 64 | 64 |
| 60 min. | | 84 | 72 | 68 | 68 | 68 | 68 | | | | | | | |
| 90 min. | | 84 | 72 | 68 | 68 | 68 | 68 | | | | | | | |
| LUNCH | | 84 | 68 | 68 | 68 | 68 | 68 | | 60 | 76 | 70 | 70 | 66 | 66 |
| 30 min. | | 84 | 76 | 72 | 72 | 68 | 68 | | 66 | 78 | 74 | 68 | 70 | 68 |
| 60 min. | | 84 | 68 | 68 | 68 | 68 | 68 | | | | | | | |
| 90 min. | | 84 | 72 | 68 | 68 | 68 | 68 | | | | | | | |
| DINNER | | 72 | 68 | 68 | 68 | 68 | 68 | | 68 | 76 | 84 | 68 | 70 | 68 |
| 30 min. | | 76 | 76 | 72 | 72 | 68 | 68 | | 70 | 80 | 80 | 70 | 66 | 66 |
| 60 min. | | 72 | 68 | 72 | 68 | 68 | 68 | | | | | | | |
| 90 min. | | 72 | 68 | 68 | 68 | 68 | 68 | | | | | | | |
| RET. | | 72 | 68 | 68 | 68 | 68 | 68 | | 74 | 64 | 78 | 66 | 64 | 64 |
| | | | | | | | | | N | H | | | | |

BR—before rising          day 3, period begins:          day 7, period ends
                          N—nausea                       H—severe headache

Such cases as these are exceptionally easy of interpretation, each being allergic to only one excitant, tobacco and ovarian hormones respectively.

A.M. (victim of multiple sclerosis) smoked a cigarette and his pulse rose from 84 to 95 in five minutes. He stopped his smoking on the zero day and the lowest daily maximum of his pulse (68) was reached on the fifth day; on which day he was able to play baseball, for the first time in months. 68 remained his *normal* maximum.

Mrs. K., age 34, suffered frequent attacks of migraine. After she began to avoid citrus fruit, her only pulse-accelerating food, her migraine occurred only at the menstrual periods. In the present instance the maximal pulse rate returned to its normal (68) on the 9th day. The pulse record on her zero day was the same as that on the 10th day.

## Interpretation of the Pulse-Record

Since the pulse began to be used as a specific indicator of the allergic causes of ill health, the "pulse-record" has come to mean the record of pulse counts made either 14 times daily on the regular three-meal schedule or at about half-hour intervals throughout the day on hourly small feedings of single foods.

The interpretation of the record of this simple procedure is often complicated by non-dietary factors, some of which have been first suspected through the experience of observant patients. One young married couple recently reported marked pulse-reactions following "sniff-tests" of wood stored in their cellar and of the unfinished under-surfaces of tables.

A marked pulse-rise occurring after rising in the morning but *before* breakfast usually points to a sensitivity to some ingredient (perfume?) of toilet articles (shaving cream or lotion). One man was found to be allergic *only* to the menthol in the "nose drops" which he used in the morning.

Women are not infrequently allergic to their own ovarian hormones which are most active at the menstrual periods or half-way between the periods: Marked symptoms and pulse acceleration occurring at those times suggest a hormone sensitivity.

Rarely, an unlucky person is found allergic to an unidentified something in the particular house in which he is living, and obtains complete relief by merely moving to another house in the same neighborhood.

Sensitivity to fresh newsprint (papers, magazines, carbon paper) can frustrate one's effort until it is discovered.

Evidently, every one affected by the newly discovered idioblaptic disease must become his own personal "allergy-detective."

It is intended here to present a few instructive pulse-records of idioblaptic persons whose illnesses were "cured" by mere avoidance of their pulse-accelerating allergens. These cases were all relatively easily solved, nearly always through interpretation of the first records.

The first two tables, 1a and 1b, are taken from my monograph, "Familial Nonreaginic Food-Allergy." (Page 100, case 8, Tables XIIa and XIIb.)

The patient Mrs. E. E., age 32, was a fully occupied housewife with a six-year old daughter. She had to care for a bedridden aunt. Her chief complaint was an annoying eruption about her mouth and chin.

## Table 1a

Pulse record on Mrs. E. E. on an unrestricted diet.

| | May 11 | May 12 | May 13 | May 15 | May 17 | May 19 | May 20 |
|---|---|---|---|---|---|---|---|
| Before rising | 61 | 57 | 64 | 56 | — | 70 | 66 |
| BREAKFAST (pulse) | 68 | 70 | 70 | 69 | 75 | 74 | 68 |
| 30' | 75 | 74 | 73 | 78 | 71 | 74 | 76 |
| 60' | 80 | 78 | 76 | 75 | 71 | 77 | 73 |
| 90' | 76 | 71 | 81 | 73 | 62 | 72 | 68 |
| DIET— | orange, coffee, wheat-cereal | pineapple, bacon, egg, bread, coffee, crab-apple jelly | apricot, bread, wheat-cereal, crab-apple jelly, coffee | applesauce, cinnamon-toast, coffee, sugar | wheat-cereal, coffee, (fudge) | egg, grapefruit, wheat-cereal, apple-butter, coffee | egg, coffee, coffee-cake |
| LUNCH | — | 75 | 69 | 68 | 80 | 68 | 74 |
| 30' | — | 89 | 65 | — | — | 76 | — |
| 60' | — | 75 | 74 | 78 | — | 78 | — |
| 90' | 69 | 71 | 82 | — | — | 74 | — |
| DIET— | macaroni, tomato, beef, cucumber, vinegar, pepper, potato, butter, coffee | chicken, noodle, tuna fish, milk, bread, lettuce, mayonnaise, olives, chocolate, pickle | tomato, potato, carrot, peas, cake, cream wine | clam chowder, liverwurst | tomato, cheese, rye-bread, tea, cheese-cake | chicken, rice, cream-cheese, apple-butter, tea | beef, potato, tomato, tea, chocolate-pudding, marshmallow |
| DINNER | 65 | 70 | 60 | 65 | 64 | 76 | 66 |
| 30' | 69 | 73 | 64 | 66 | 68 | 78 | 68 |
| 60' | 68 | 74 | 68 | 84 | 68 | 75 | 66 |
| 90' | 63 | 69 | 62 | 65 | 64 | 72 | — |
| DIET— | tuna fish, olive, tomato, celery, potato, mayonnaise, apple-juice | lamb, potato, barley, beets, pineapple, walnut-cake | beef, potato, milk, spinach, peach-cake, cinnamon, coffee, sugar | ham, potato, carrot, apple, peach-cream cake, coffee | mackerel, potato, tea, tomato, ice cream | beef, corn, potato, coffee, chocolate-pudding, marshmallow | |

## Table 1b
### Pulse record on Mrs. E. E. on selected diet.

| | May 29 | May 30 | May 31 | June 1 | June 2 |
|---|---|---|---|---|---|
| | pulse | pulse | pulse | pulse | pulse |
| Before rising | | 60 | 58 | 58 | 60 |
| BREAKFAST | | 66 | 68 | 67 | 68 |
| 30' | | 67 | 60 | 69 | 68 |
| 60' | | 70 | 62 | 70 | — |
| 90' | | 66 | 61 | 68 | — |
| DIET — | | pep-cereal, coffee, bread | pep-cereal, coffee, sugar, bread | pep-cereal, coffee, cake | wheat-cereal, coffee |
| LUNCH | 62 | 64 | 66 | 64 | — |
| 30' | 65 | 66 | 66 | 66 | — |
| 60' | 68 | 69 | 68 | 68 | — |
| 90' | 66 | 68 | 70 | 64 | — |
| DIET — | apple, lettuce, mayonnaise | beef, potato, carrot, onion, corn, coffee, apple-pie | lettuce, bread, sardines, mayonnaise, rice, apple-juice | carrot, beet, lettuce, mayonnaise, apple-juice | |
| DINNER | 66 | 64 | 66 | 64 | 66 |
| 30' | 62 | 62 | 68 | 68 | 68 |
| 60' | 64 | 64 | 68 | 66 | 68 |
| 90' | 60 | 60 | 66 | 64 | 64 |
| DIET — | beef, potato, corn, coffee, apple-pie | lamb, tomato, potato, coffee, apple | tomato, lamb, potato, beets, coffee | ham, potato, carrot, apple, mayonnaise, coffee | beef, carrot, pepper, lettuce, potato, applesauce, coffee, mayonnaise |
| RETIRING | 60 | 58 | 60 | 60 | 62 |

Table 1a was made following a ten minute verbal instruction. There was no consultation between May 11 and May 20, when the record was received.

Interpretation of such an original record *regularly begins with the noting of the lowest and highest counts,* which in this instance were 56 and 89—a range of 33 beats. The maximal normal range of the human pulse rate is *16 beats,* hence the observed range of 33 indicates that E. E. is allergic.

If we take 12 beats provisionally as her *normal* range, her normal maximum would be about 68. On this basis if the pulse did not rise above 68 after a large meal, it could be assumed that no allergenic foods were eaten at that meal. It is seen that all the "dinners" of May 11, 13, 17, and 20 qualified in that respect. The patient therefore was instructed to limit her diet through five days to the combined list of items from the four dinners—which she did.

Table 1b was made through most of five days on the restricted diet and under otherwise the same conditions of physical and psychological "stress" that had prevailed throughout the ten days of the preliminary tests.

The low and high counts of table 1b are 58 and 70 respectively, a range of 12, which can be normal. Also the high count is *exactly* reached on each of the three days on which the full 14 counts were made. It should be noted by the beginner that a single count of 71 should have aroused suspicion of exposure to an inhaled allergic excitant, to be watched for thereafter.

The record teaches the highly important lesson that the *normal* pulse is not affected by *ordinary* physical activity nor by the psychological influences, nor by digestion of nonallergenic foods.

E. E. continued the testing of other foods, looking for

any that would elevate her pulse above the normal maximum 70, but she found none. Her facial eruption soon healed.

Looking back, it can be seen that the foods which affected the pulse at breakfast on May 11, 12, 13 and 15 were respectively orange, pineapple, apricot and cinnamon.

Tables 2 and 3 are taken from my report in the Spanish journal of allergy, *Alergologia* No. 20.

Table 2 is that of Mr. J. R. B., age 74, whose eczematoid condition of his legs had resisted local "treatments" for ten years. He lived alone in a scantily furnished house. The pulse-test with cigar was negative. He avoided the cabbage family and onion, having himself found that they caused migraine headache.

It is seen that the *low* count in the four days from June 4 to 7 was 60, the highest 68—a range of 8 beats, which could be normal. This result showed that he was not allergic to any food that he ate in the four days. The record gave no indication of a sensitivity to house-dust; yet the exclusion of food and tobacco sensitivity compelled a suspicion of the third *most likely* allergen, the ubiquitous and almost unavoidable "house-dust."

And so his meager furniture, rugs and bedding were Dust-Sealed as a conclusive test, on a hot, sunny June day on his lawn. They were quite dry a few hours later and could be replaced in the late afternoon.

Mr. B slept on his Dust-Sealed bed mattress that night, and in the morning for the first time found his pulse four beats lower than ever before. His maximum rate also dropped four beats and this lower level was indefinitely maintained.

*Table 2*

Showing the drop of the pulse-rate following the use of "Dust Seal" in the case of a severe eczematoid eruption, caused by sensitivity to "House-Dust." (See chapter 9.)

*Pulse rate*

| June | 4 | 5 | 6 | 7 |
|---|---|---|---|---|
| Before rising | 64 | 60 | 60 | 60 |
| Maximum | 68 | 68 | 68 | 68 |
| Retiring | 64 | 60 | 64 | 60 |

June 8, bed-mattress and furniture treated with "Dust-Seal"

| June | 9 | 10 | 11 | 12 |
|---|---|---|---|---|
| Before rising | 56 | 56 | 56 | 56 |
| Maximum | 64 | 64 | 64 | 64 |
| Retiring | 60 | 60 | 60 | 60 |

The pulse was counted 14 times each day; just before each meal, three times after each meal at half-hour intervals, just before retiring and before rising in the morning.

The eczema was practically healed in two months and there has been no recurrence in the past seven years.

Table No. 3 is that of Mr. W., whose brief case-history is recounted on pages 124-5 of this book. His chief symptom was daily, painless vomiting.

Most beginners, on being handed this record, first scan the list of foods, looking for a likely cause of the frequent vomiting. The reader has, by this time, learned to look first at the figures of the pulse-counts, where he will find the answer. The low count is 70, the highest is 80, a range of 10, which can be normal.

This observation, by itself, shows that Mr. W. was not allergic to any of the foods he had been eating; his vomiting was *not* due to a food sensitivity.

Most idioblaptic allergies are due to some food-sensitivity. The next most commonly incriminated aller-

# THE PULSE TEST

## Table 3

Mr. W., ship's purser, suddenly suffered abdominal pain with frequent painless vomiting in November.

January 5.
A.M.   Pulse
10:45 — 74 — before rising
                begin smoking
11:00 — 74 — coffee, sugar,
                cream
P.M.

1:00 — 80 — coffee, sugar,
                cream
2:00 — 76
2:30 — 78 — grapes cheese
3:30 — 73
7:00 — 70 — ham, bread,
                butter, cheese,
                tomato, lettuce,
                mayonnaise,
                pepper
8:00 vomited
        75
8:35 — 74
9:15 — 72 — coffee, sugar,
                milk, pie,
                chocolate
11:30 — 70

P.M.
2:00 — 80
2:15 — 76 — veal, potato,
                beans, pork,
                tomato,
                cucumber,
                lettuce, tapioca,
                sugar, cream,
                coffee
3:00 — 74
    vomited
3:45 — 80
5:30 — 78 — doughnuts, coffee
5:45 vomited
6:00 — 74
6:30 — 72
7:40 — 75 — cheese-sandwich,
                lemon soda,
                brandy
9:45 — 78
10:15 — 72
11:10 — 72
11:30 — 72 — coffee, sugar
    vomited
12:00 — 72

January 6.
A.M.                    Pulse
3:00 — 74 — retired
8:30 — 70 — before rising
                began smoking
9:00 — 74 — bacon, egg,
                biscuits, coffee,
                sugar
    vomited
9:30 — 76
10:00 — 80

January 7.
A.M.   Pulse
1:00 — 70 — before retiring
9:30 — 74 — before rising
                began smoking
9:45 — 74 — coffee, sugar

gen is tobacco which affects about three-fourths of the population (Granvill F. Knight). Mr. W. smoked constantly through the day from the time he rose in the morning.

The allergic pulse-reaction to tobacco has been found regularly to occur within 15 minutes after the individual begins to smoke, and fortunately Mr. W. always recorded his pulse just before smoking and 15 minutes later. Thus on January 5 his pulse at 10.45 A.M. "before smoking" was 72 and at 11:00 it was 74, which was well within his normal range. Again, on January 7, at 9.30 before smoking his pulse was 74 and 15 minutes later it was still 74. Therefore Mr. W. is not allergic to tobacco. These dependably negative tests of food and tobacco leave "house-dust" as the most likely suspect as the specific cause of the vomiting. In fact the record contains significant data pointing to dust-sensitivity. Let us examine these data.

We find that the pulse-record says "Not guilty" to foods and tobacco. However, note that the low count does not occur always "before rising" after the night's rest. This permits a *suspicion* of dust-sensitivity (rule 7).

The explanation of this phenomenon is a little involved. First, the phenomenon can occur only in the absence of the reactions of common food-sensitivities and reactions to tobacco smoke; because these are relatively strong "major" allergens, whereas dust-sensitivity is nearly, if not quite always a weak or "minor" one. Secondly, the dust-allergen is generally 10 or 20 times more concentrated in used bed-mattresses than it is in rugs and carpets. Thus the exposure to "dust" while in bed can be greater than it is elsewhere in a house that is not Dust-Sealed.

Mr. W.'s "before rising" pulse on Jan. 5 was not 70 but 72; and on Jan. 7, his pulse before retiring was 70 (his lowest), but it had risen to 74 as he was resting after the night's sleep.

Mr. W. accepted the interpretation, Dust-Sealed his apartment and purser's quarters and was immediately and permanently relieved of his distressing condition, which, by the way, had been classed as "psychosomatic" in two Marine hospitals.

The following tentative rules of technic and interpretation of the pulse-dietary record may be helpful to those who are beginners in the art. One must not, however, forget the occasional exceptions to these rules.

*Rule 1.* If your pulse-count taken standing is greater than that taken sitting, this is a positive indication of present "allergic tension" (Sanchez-Cuenca).

*Rule 2.* If at least 14 pulse-counts are being made each day, and if your daily maximal pulse-rate is constant (within one or two beats) for three days in succession, this indicates that all "food-allergens" have been avoided on those days.

*Rule 3.* If your daily maximal pulse-rate varies more than two beats; for example, Monday 72, Tuesday 78, Wednesday 76, Thursday 61, you are certainly allergic, provided there is no infection.

*Rule 4.* If the ingestion of a frequently eaten food causes no acceleration of your pulse (at least 6 beats above your estimated normal maximum) that food can be tentatively considered non-allergenic for you.

*Rule 5.* If exposure to "house-dust" causes irregularity of your pulse, this regularly excludes the commonly eaten foods as allergens, since "housedust" is, at least usually, a "minor" allergen; hence it does not affect persons who are protected by the stronger reactions that would be caused by foods.

*Rule 6.* Your pulse-reaction to an inhaled allergen (particularly "house-dust") is more likely to be of short duration than that to a major food allergen.

*Rule 7.* Pulse-rates that are not more than 6 beats above the estimated normal daily maximum should not be blamed on a recently eaten food but on an inhalant or a recurrent reaction.

*Rule 8.* If your minimum pulse-rate does not regularly occur "before rising," after the night's rest, but at some other time in the day, this usually indicates sensitivity to the "house-dust" in mattresses or pillows.

*Rule 9.* If you are not susceptible to common colds, you are probably allergic to only few, if any, commonly eaten foods; though you may be allergic to some inhaled substances, for example "house-dust" which may even cause *respiratory* symptoms.

Now I come to an interesting point.

Good intentions are not enough if you are serious about discovering the cause of your ill health, present or future.

You *must* decide to devote yourself to pulse counting for the required number of days.

It all seems simple. And yet I know people who are bedridden with nothing but time on their hands, who would not devote the time and energy necessary to complete a survey.

I know automobile owners who, if told they were pouring a corrosive chemical into their car engines when they used a specific type of gasoline, would spend days testing the truth of my statement. But these same people if told that they are pouring what are to them poisons into their own body engines, would not take one hour to test the truth of my statement.

For five or ten days of testing, you may be rewarded with five or ten years, or more, of additional illness-free life-span.

You are being given a roadmap to the fountain of youth. Use it.

Incidentally, you *must* give up smoking immediately, at least for the duration of these tests. Cigarettes are a major killer. At least 300,000 deaths each year are attributed to cigarette smoking. I believe this is half the actual number, for thousands die from secondary smoking (inhaling other people's smoke) and for reasons falsely blamed on other causes.

# (4)

# Your Heart and Your Pulse

Your heart is a personal matter; as personal as your diary or your income-tax report. Its beat can explain how you look, act and feel. If its pattern is right, life can be a joyful, pleasant experience. If its pattern is wrong, life can be a weary drudgery, fraught with headaches, constipation, and so many of other illnesses we have mentioned.

You shouldn't wear your heart on your sleeve, but you should get acquainted with it by feeling your pulse beneath your sleeve.

Incidentally, much is known about heart damage, but that knowledge does little good to the seemingly healthy man or woman who keels over dead with a heart attack. Almost everyone knows of one case where death came unexpectedly and "apparently without cause" from a sudden heart attack.

So-called "heart attacks" claim at least 600,000 victims in this country each year.

Since there is no way to foretell whether you are destined to be among next year's thousands, you may be curious to understand how a heart-attack occurs. Here is the pertinent life-story of one typical case.

Soon after he was born Mr. X. became allergic to milk and to tobacco smoke. However, neither of these substances affected his health noticeably, although his medical acquaintances remarked upon his fast and irregular pulse due, they thought, to his "strenuous life."

"Coming of age," he began to smoke "heavily" in spite of vague suspicions that smoking was not "good for him." His blood pressure was always normal.

At the age of 45, with no premonition whatever, he suddenly fell to the floor in his office in a heart-attack, which completely incapacitated him for two years, after which time a second major attack carried him off.

In this man the heart was the most important organ which was to become *susceptible* to his allergic reactions. However, the local susceptibility was not *established* in him till he reached the age of 45. If he had stopped smoking and avoided milk one week previous to the date of his attack, the attack would not have occurred. The heart *had not been damaged* by his long indulgence in his allergens. But after the critical age of the cardiac susceptibility had been reached, a resumption of smoking at any time would have been quickly followed by the allergic catastrophe. This had happened in one of my cases.

The allergically fast pulse is caused by an allergic reaction in the nervous system controlling the heart beat, which does not directly affect the heart muscle. The rapid pulse of allergy does no lasting harm, even after many years. It is the local susceptibility of the blood vessels that nourish the *heart muscle* which is responsible for a heart attack.

You owe it to your heart then to learn how it is behaving. And if it is beating too fast, you owe it to yourself to learn why, and to remove the cause of that too-fast beat or acceleration *in time.*

The first question from an allergic person seeking relief through the pulse-dietary survey is usually. "How fast should my heart beat; what is my normal rate?"

To this there is only one answer, "That cannot be determined with certainty until at least four or five days after you have begun to avoid *all* of your dietary and other allergens (tobacco, dust, fumes, perfumes, et cetera)."

As I have said earlier, the reason for this is that there is a great variation of normal pulse-rate among different individuals. Some text books still state that the normal pulse-rate is about 72 beats per minute, but the truth is there is no "normal" pulse-rate.

Consider in its course over a sufficient period (possibly a week is enough), the normal person's pulse may be sufficiently individualized to be as unique in its character as are the finger-prints. And there is no "normal" finger-print.

The pulse-character is expressed for practical diagnostic purpose in its general level (low or medium or high), and in its daily range (interval between the lowest number of beats per minute and the highest number of beats per minute). Other things that may be individual are possibly variations in the daily minimal low and maximal high rates, although the latter are constant enough (not varying more than two beats per minute) to serve as dependable indicators of the success of the dietary course.

I mean that when the patient's *maximal* pulse-rate has been brought, by a selection of diet, to a variation from day to day of not more than two beats per minute, the survey has been successful, and the allergic symptoms should have disappeared. There are rare exceptions to this rule.

Gross differences of the pulse-character are found in different nonallergic persons when the pulse is counted fourteen times daily for two to five days.

|  | Lowest count | Highest count | Range |
|---|---|---|---|
| 1 | 62 | 72 | 10 |
| 2 | 62 | 72 | 10 |
| 3 | 66 | 76 | 10 |
| 4 | 69 | 76 | 7 |
| 5 | 70 | 78 | 8 |
| 6 | 72 | 80 | 8 |
| 7 | 72 | 82 | 10 |
| Average | 68 | 76.5 | 9 |

The table above shows the essential data obtained from seven pupil nurses, all of whom, as well as their parents, were free from allergic symptoms. It is seen that although the highest count of nurse 7 was greater than that of nurse 1, the range from low to high was the same in both—10.

It is astonishing to learn through the report of Dr. George C. Deaver of New York University that the outstanding runners, Leslie MacMitchell, Glenn Cunningham and Paavo Nurmi had the low pulse-rates of 38,

42, and 47 respectively. Although such low rates are unusual—among 104 persons, I encountered only four with minimal rates below 50—they are found in perfectly healthy people; they are not abnormal.

The range of the pulse varies greatly in different normal individuals. This is illustrated in the table (on pages 70–71) showing a survey of fifty persons. All of these people had been brought out of their various allergic miseries, as you may be, through the pulse-dietary method.

The one patient, a man of 30 years, with the range of only two beats, regularly reported a count of 60 taken before rising in the morning. As soon as he was up the count was 62, and remained at that rate throughout his busy work-day, irrespective of his meals—so long as he avoided his pulse-accelerating foods. During the past ten years in which he has adhered to this regime he has been free from his allergic symptoms, including the major one, epileptic seizures. Previously his pulse-rate had ranged from 78 to 102.

The dependability of the pulse as an indicator of allergic reaction is illustrated in the case of C. G., age 15, whose symptoms were chronic urticaria (hives), recurring headache, abnormal tiredness, occasional dizziness and "canker sores."

It was the urticaria that annoyed her most, both physically and cosmetically, and drove her to the tedium of the daily 22 pulse counts. Her normal range was found to be unusually low—52 to 61; the sole cause of her hives was wheat, and there were only two other food allergens, strawberry and beef.

*Range of the Pulse-Rate in Fifty Food-Allergic Persons Before and After Dietary Treatment*

| Patient | Sex | Age | Range of Pulse-Rate | |
| --- | --- | --- | --- | --- |
| | | | After Treatment | At Start of Treatment |
| E. F. C. | M | 49 | 68 – 80 | to    180 |
| A. F. C. | F | 65 | 58 – 70 | 66 – 100 |
| M. M. D. | F | 27 | 70 – 80 | 70 – 100 |
| A. R. | M | 28 | 70 – 84 | 66 – 108 |
| C. T. | M | 26 | 72 – 78 | 65 – 112 |
| J. G. | F | 36 | 66 – 80 | 66 – 100 |
| H. E.* | F | 49 | 58 – 76 | 76 – 106 |
| W. W. F. | M | 57 | 56 – 68 | 66 – 100 |
| M. W. F. | M | 52 | 58 – 72 | 72 – 100 |
| A. W. F. | M | 17 | 60 – 72 | 70 – 90 |
| F. C. F. | F | 16 | 58 – 70 | 58 – 84 |
| M. B. | M | 22 | 64 – 76 | 64 – 100 |
| P. W. | F | 47 | 62 – 78 | 68 – 100 |
| R. M. | F | 22 | 62 – 78 | 68 – 100 |
| A. P. | M | 70 + | 70 – 74 | 72 – 100 |
| S. I. H. | M | 40 | 68 – 80 | 68 – 108 |
| H. A. S. | M | 58 | 60 – 74 | 60 – 105 |
| J. F. | F | 53 | 68 – 80 | 68 – 108 |
| W. S. C.* | M | 41 | 46 – 62 | 46 – 70 |
| J. V.* | F | 34 | 48 – 64 | 44 – 78 |
| E. B. | M | 50 | 72 – 76 | 82 – 108 |
| Dr. R. | F | 26 | 70 – 76 | 70 – 90 |
| R. F. | F | 34 | 62 – 76 | 64 – 114 |
| A. F. | F | 10 | 74 – 78 | 82 – 124 |
| N. V. W. | M | 38 | 62 – 76 | 64 – 86 |
| Dr. I. P.* | F | 46 | 72 – 78 | 84 – 104 |
| L. H. B. | M | 20 | 58 – 70 | 60 – 90 |
| J. J. V. | F | 38 | 62 – 74 | 70 – 94 |
| C. B. | M | 23 | 67 – 72 | 72 – 100 |
| K. S. | F | 48 | 70 – 80 | 70 – 110 |
| M. D. B. | F | 50 + | 52 – 60 | 62 – 90 |
| G. H. | F | 17 | 54 – 66 | 66 – 102 |
| E. K. | F | 27 | 58 – 66 | 60 – 96 |

| Patient | Sex | Age | Range of Pulse-Rate | |
|---------|-----|-----|---------------------|---|
| | | | After Treatment | At Start of Treatment |
| A. S. | F | 50 | 62 – 76 | 66 – 96 |
| J. K | M | 30 | 60 – 62 | 78 – 102 |
| G. B. | F | 55 | 64 – 74 | 64 – 92 |
| J. B. | M | 35 | 68 – 78 | 68 – 100 |
| O. W. L. | M | 52 | 68 – 80 | 70 – 98 |
| Mrs. E. B. | F | 36 | 48 – 60 | 47 – 79 |
| M. P. | F | 11 | 60 – 72 | 74 – 116 |
| M. S. | F | 31 | 64 – 74 | 64 – 100 |
| W. G. | F | 21 | 66 – 78 | 66 – 86 |
| L. S. | M | 24 | 56 – 68 | 56 – 88 |
| B. B. | M | 20 | 58 – 68 | 58 – 78 |
| T. C. F. | M | 50 | 54 – 68 | 54 – 90 |
| E. H. | M | 50 | 60 – 68 | 66 – 88 |
| C. A. E. | M | 50 | 60 – 68 | 66 – 90 |
| E. A. | F | 63 | 56 – 68 | 75 – 100 |
| A. C. M. | F | 50 | 64 – 78 | 62 – 100 |
| G. C. N. | M | 55 | 70 – 78 | 74 – 88 |

*These patients did not complete the dietary diagnosis and undoubtedly are mildly affected by unidentified minor allergens, although completely relieved of their major symptoms.

Wheat was suspected on the second day, and thereafter avoided, but the hives and the elevated pulse continued for two and a half days.

Beef was then tested (highest count 84), and caused no hives, but affected the pulse in the subsequent six days! (The daily highest counts were 67, 72, 67, 65 and 62). Then followed six days in which the count reached 61 (only 60 on one day), but no higher excepting the tests with strawberry in which it reached 66 and 67 respectively (a very feeble sensitivity). The low count on all those six days was 52.

Then she retested wheat at breakfast, and in 30

minutes the pulse registered 90, remaining between 74 and 88 the rest of the day. After lunch she reported "covered with hives; face swollen." The eruption persisted through the next two days.

Here we have a physically active, popular honor student, too busy to be neurotic, yet presenting some of the common symptoms of neurasthenia, which lacked only the mental depression that would logically ensue if the condition should continue so long that it would seem incurable.

In the first two days of her test the sole cause of all her troubles was detected, and there has been no recurrence of them in the subsequent four years excepting a mild swelling of the face (sufficient warning for a young woman) after incautious nibbling at pastry.

The pulse is sometimes affected by menstruation but, so far as I have had opportunity to observe, only in *allergic* women.

Not all allergic women exhibit this effect and, in some who do there is no other disturbance at the periods. However, some women suffer at the periods not only a rapid heart beat, but also typical allergic symptoms (migraine, bronchial asthma, constipation). Assuming a particular excitant of such allergic manifestations one can only imagine that it is produced in unusually large quantity in the female generative organs at a certain time in the menstrual cycle.

Mrs. M. M., age 40, mother of two young children, both allergic, is a sufferer from bronchial asthma. The preliminary pulse-dietary survey revealed no "food allergens," but the pulse record over several months pointed to an internal allergen that caused severe, indeed alarming, continued asthma in the early stages of each of three periods.

The patient could not recall the circumstances of the earlier periods. The pulse in these attacks ranged well over 100. On one of these occasions she required injections of epinephrine throughout one night. It was decided to induce premature menopause with X-ray (ten spaced treatments). There were two periods after the treatments, both accompanied with high pulse (up to 104), but with milder asthma. Then the periods ceased, and also the asthmatic crises and the rapid pulse.

Mrs. L. P., age 25, was subject to abnormal tiredness and constipation. The pulse-dietary survey revealed only two excitants, tobacco and the microorganisms in cheese (yeast, bacteria). She was not allergic to milk. Smoking elevated the pulse from 64 to 80 in five minutes. Avoidance of her allergens was followed by relief of her symptoms between the periods, but both the tiredness and the constipation were present for a few days at or just previous to the periods.

Mrs. E. B., age 36, had long suffered from daily nausea and vomiting. Her weight was about 90 pounds, height five feet. The pulse-dietary survey, controlled in correspondence (I have never seen her) revealed sensitivity to a number of important foods; cereals, milk, potato, pork, fish, fowl, cane sugar, peanut and banana. Her acute symptoms ceased immediately upon avoidance of all her "food-poisons" and slowly thereafter, upon her greatly restricted diet, she gained weight up to 120 pounds.

This patient never suffers allergic symptoms at the

periods, but a menstrual allergic effect is registered upon the pulse-rate. Curiously this effect is not always an acceleration, which is usual, but is sometimes a moderate slowing of the rate. Such a symptomless allergic pulse-reaction is sometimes due to external allergens. Indeed, it is well known that a victim of high blood pressure (which is usually allergic) may die suddenly in a stroke or heart attack in active middle life without ever having been "sick a day."

It is well known to physicians that the child's pulse tends to be faster than the adult pulse. However, this difference is seen only in those individuals in the two respective groups showing rates below that which is certainly allergic.

This is clearly seen in a survey of the pulse-rates that were taken in two groups of children one hour after lunch. Among 50 between the ages of 8 and 10 only two (4 percent) showed a rate of 76 or less; whereas among 65 who had passed puberty (14 to 17) 21 (33 percent) showed rates of 76 or less. On the other hand, about half of each group showed rates of 90 or more, which in most instances indicates the presence of the allergic constitution.

The maximal pulse-rate in the normal nonallergic child has been the same, in my limited experience, as that in the normal adult—84.

It is my belief that there is nothing more valuable that you can do for your child than to learn the secrets of his heart through his pulse, and to teach him to join you in avoiding those things to which he is personally allergic.

For then you will be giving your child the gift of good health, and what other gift can cause so much long-time happiness, and pay such pleasant dividends?

# (5)

# "That Tired Feeling"

For a purely philosophical purpose, which will become apparent presently, I think of the bodily functions as divided into two main groups; the active and the passive.

By the "active" functions I mean those of motion, of the senses, of alimentation, of reproduction, of the mental processes, and of another which I feel unable to define, and which I shall call the spiritual function.

By the "passive" functions I mean such as those concerned in the protection of the individual against injurious influences—functions exercised by the covering of the body with its appendages (hair, nails), the nerves of pain-, heat-, and cold-perception, and the bony skeleton.

A noteworthy fact has escaped the attention of many of us because of our inherited physical disabilities, and that is that the *healthful* exercise of each of the normal functions of the active group is attended with a specific pleasure and usually with a general sense of well-being.

My special medical experience has convinced me that if the exercise of any active function is not pleasurable, this is either because that function has not been healthfully used, or because it is subject to some abnormal condition—usually of allergic nature.

The protracted disuse of an active function results not only in a sacrifice of pleasure, but in positive discomfort or pain, and a gradual loss of the function. (The outstanding exception here is the reproductive function, the disuse of which is often punished with discomfort, pain and other disorders, but not with its loss). The active bodily functions, then, are intended to be used, and their healthful use in the *normal* body is rewarded with a pleasure that frequently fulfills our concepts of human happiness.

In passing I should take note of the well-known fact that the pleasures of the listed active functions are not equal; that those of the spiritual function, which so often involve a renunciation of those lower ones of the order known as sensual, are the ones that are reserved for the reward of the highest aspirations of mankind. It may be useful to some to observe that there is no inherent incompatibility in the enjoyment of the pleasures of *all* of the active functions to their healthful maximums; there seems to be no moral profit in the self-deprivation *per se* of the pleasure of any active function.

Against the background of the foregoing considerations we examine tiredness and fatigue.

By normal tiredness I mean the physically perceptible consequences of prolonged but not necessarily excessive physical exertion. It is not unpleasant and indeed it arouses anticipations of the pleasures of relaxation and of "gentle sleep." On the other hand, all of us are acquainted with the difference between the tiredness of physical exertion, and that resulting for example from muscular disuse. Many are familiar with the physical refreshment that vigorous sport can bring to replace the weariness of a day's confinement in a sedentary occupation.

A prominent feature of the function of motion is the pleasure in its normal exercise; the urge to use the muscular system is seen in the act of "stretching" in both man and animal. And so the normal man, after a day of the healthful use of his active functions and a healthful interval of rest and motionless sleep, wakes in the morning, obeys the urge to stretch his muscles and sinews from fingers to toes and springs out of bed, filled with the pleasant anticipation of the exercise of his refreshed and recharged body.

He is irked by inactivity; may welcome an excuse to run; prefers walking reasonable distances rather than riding; climbs stairs rather than wait for the elevator; and spends his vacations in unaccustomed, sometimes exhausting physical activity, deliberately depriving himself of the comforts and conveniences of his regular way of living. It is seen that normal tiredness is the natural result of the use of the function of motion. A proper synonym of tiredness of this kind is "fatigue."

"Abnormal tiredness" on the contrary is not a result of the use of any bodily function; it does not express a need for rest; there is no pleasure in it—indeed it is characteristically an unpleasant, often painful phenomenon, it is fequently most marked upon waking from a long sleep—not a consequence of sleep but present *in spite* of the rest. Abnormal tiredness is regularly associated with common allergic symptoms, especially migraine and lesser grades of recurrent headache, but in itself it may constitute the chief complaint of an adult subject.

It should always be suspected as the cause of "laziness" in children or in adults. In other words, laziness should be looked upon as a sign of an underlying physical abnormality to be treated not psychologically, but medically through identification and avoidance of its causes. "Reasoning" with a lethargic child is exactly as reasonable as chiding a victim of polio for his awkward gait.

Abnormal tiredness is one of the most common symptoms of "food-allergy," standing close to headache in this respect. Its allergic nature is attested by the fact that the symptom vanished in all of the 56 cases herein reported on, after avoidance of all of the "food-allergens." A common report from the patients was "I feel like a new person."

For the question: How does "food-allergy" cause the abnormal tiredness? the following facts may provide an answer:

Wherever it is possible to examine the local effects (lesion) of "food-allergy" this is often seen to consist in an abnormal outflow of fluid (dilute plasma) from the small terminal blood vessels into the tissue where the fluid is prevented from a normal return to the circulation— through the lymph channels—by some obstruction, which is an essential part of the allergic process.

Thus a swelling under pressure develops in the affected area which is easily seen in hives, nasal allergy (sinusitis), asthma and glaucoma.

The allergic fluid is often distributed widely throughout the body,* and at the close of an attack this fluid may be suddenly eliminated in great quantity through the kidneys.

After all your "food allergens" have been identified and avoided, and the allergic symptoms have disappeared, a sudden considerable and permanent loss of weight may be experienced. This ranges in some cases between five and fifteen pounds. Thus you have a measure of the general water-logging of the body, and with it one reasonable explanation of the symptom of abnormal tiredness.

In some cases showing a condition of overweight the first rapid loss of weight is followed, for a few weeks, by a slower loss to a point where irrespective of the amount of food eaten the weight remains indefinitely constant. This slower decrease of weight presumably represents a loss of excessive fat.

On the other hand, some fool-allergic persons come for anti-allergic treatment in a state of malnutrition having loss weight on account of their allergic indigestion (daily vomiting, for example, or gastric pain or "poor appetite"). These persons in time regain their normal weight, sometimes in spite of a sharp restriction of their diet entailed by the avoidance of their "food-poisons."

One obtains an impression from these repeated experiences that overweight is probably not due primarily to overeating, but in most instances is a consequence—directly, and possibly also indirectly through a disturbance of some glands of internal secretion (hormones)—of "food-allergy." It should be pointed out that despite

*Von Pirquet and Schick: *Serum Sickness.*

insurance company claims to the contrary, the *normal* range of human body-weight in relation to age and height has not been ascertained.

Returning from this digression to our stated topic, we recognize the term "abnormal tiredness" as a misnomer. It is not fatigue, but the disagreeable "food-allergic" symptoms that deserve a new name, if only to remove a stigma from its victims, young and old.

I first met Lyle Stuart as a journalist. Later he launched a book publishing enterprise with this book.

When Lyle lived in North Bergen, New Jersey, he wrote scripts for the State Department's Voice of America and the American Medical Association as well as comic strip continuities. He would work at home. Often in mid-afternoon he walked a block to the local ice cream parlor and enjoyed a whipped-cream-topped butter pecan ice cream sundae.

He would walk back to his apartment. Invariably he would lie down. He felt tired. His back ached. He usually didn't do much writing for the balance of the day.

It was only when he had become familiar with the pulse-test and took it himself that he discovered (1) his normal pulse range was 60 to 78 and (2) pecans accelerated his pulse rate to the mid-90's within minutes!

He gave up pecans. The tiredness and the backaches came no more.

The victim of allergic tiredness can be a miserable person, especially if he suffers also from recurrent headaches.

Feeling a need for rest, he avoids exertion, thus adding

the real weariness of disuse of his body to his allergic discomfort until in an extreme case any exertion becomes a torture.

It is not difficult to imagine such a person turning to drink or drugs or worse, though one may suspect that such a course may be found to indicate a particular defect of "character" due conceivably to a particularly localized allergic lesion of the brain.

Every abnormality of behavior must have a cause; the means is now at hand wherewith to seek the causes due to allergy in order to control them.

It should be mentioned that the symptom of "tiredness" results sometimes from causes other than allergy; infections, which are recognizable through the associated signs, and possibly vitamin-deficiency, which is not so easily recognized. However, in my twenty-year study of inheritable food-allergy I have not encountered any instance of abnormal tiredness that could be traced with certainty to a deficiency of a particular vitamin.

# (6)

# "Almost Miraculous" Case Histories: Diabetes, Ulcers, Eczema, Hemorrhoids, Overweight, Epilepsy, Hives

This chapter is intended to point up the difference between the medical "treatment" of the symptoms of disease and the removal or avoidance of its causes. In many serious conditions the "treatment" must stop short of removal of the cause because that is not known. And so, the symptoms are treated.

Treating a symptom of a blaze will no more put out a fire than treating a disease symptom will put out the disease. If a house is on fire, it may seem helpful to put out the blaze that you can see on the roof. But the fire still smolders between the walls—and the blaze will eventually make itself known one way or the other.

Join me while I show you specifics.

The description of two of the "serious conditions," diabetes and ulcer as being of allergic nature, is being published here for the first time.

They have not been offered separately to regular medical journals for the reason that those journals have refused to print any reports involving the use of the pulse-dietary procedure.

There is too a standard objection with some medical periodicals against a report concerning only a "few" instances of successful "treatment" of previously "incurable" or intractable conditions.

The medical practitioner is thus practically relieved of the privilege of exercising his private judgment about some new ideas of the cause and prevention of chronic disease. It can be reported here that not all family physicians approve this tradition, which is equal to censorship.

## Diabetes

Diabetes is a serious disease. It has long been known that the cause of diabetes is some continual interference with the body's normal production or utilization of insulin, which goes on in the pancreas.

If you are a diabetic, your pancreas may not produce enough insulin to take care of the quantity of carbohydrate which is needed to keep you warm and active.

The discovery of insulin was a fine accomplishment. It provided a way to treat the chief *symptom* of diabetes.

However, insulin injections do not *cure* the disease. The original cause remains. It continues to act. So, in spite of the insulin, many people die of their diabetes.

I began to wonder if diabetes might be due to "food-allergy" affecting the pancreas. This thought occurred shortly after I became convinced that hypertension is caused by "food-allergy" affecting the kidney, another internal organ. Not only were my own observations convincing, but I noted similar independent observations by Dr. Sumner Price.

And then, the first two cases of diabetes came to me, and asked to be put to the tests.

Dr. and Mrs. C. wrote to me as follows:

"If you are interested in testing any theories on two diabetics with pronounced food-allergies, we would be glad to cooperate with you by serving as guinea-pigs. We don't react positively to the skin-tests, but noticed, however, that pulse and blood-pressure were normal after fasting."

To this I replied to Mrs. C., "You and Dr. C. seem to be mind-readers! I do not remember having publicly expressed the idea that diabetes may be an effect of food-allergy, but that idea has seemed to me entirely plausible."

The pulse survey revealed a number of food-sensitivities in both of them, although cereals seemed to be chief offenders. I suggested sympathectomy, but they decided to try simple elimination of the cereals.

In September, not having had word from them since July 1, I wrote for news, and received this reply from Mrs. C. "We have improved tremendously simply by doing without cereals. We use potato instead. I can tolerate *one cup of sugar* at a time. I tried it two weekends. Ran no sugar, took no insulin! My husband's insulin dosage gets lower as he improves. We look better than in years."

The "sugar-tolerance" test for diabetes is usually done by having the patient eat about a half-cup of grape sugar (glucose) at one time. If the individual is diabetic his body is not able to store up that entire amount, and the excess is thrown out through the kidneys with the urine. He "runs" sugar.

When Mrs. C. ate a whole cup of sugar at one time without taking insulin and "ran no sugar" this result proved that her pancreas had resumed its duty of insulin-production, and that the artificial assistance of injected insulin was no longer needed.

Three years later they wrote that they were still well. At that time I heard from Dr. Milo G. Meyer of his own independent control of diabetes with the use of the pulse-survey.

When I first said the foods you eat could affect the intensity of your diabetes, many laughed at me. Later, they laughed too at a fellow named Nathan Pritikin. He was more vulnerable to their laughter because he was a layman with no formal medical training.

Citizen Pritikin came to the conclusion that diet and exercise could often control diabetes. He persevered against the ridicule and the almost universal opposition of the medical profession.

What he said was correct. By eliminating certain foods from your diet—in other words by changing what you eat—you alter the course of diabetes. Nathan Pritikin advocated a high carbohydrate, low protein, very low fat diet. Such a diet, together with a structured exercise regimen, has been very effective in controlling diabetes in adults.

Initially, the medical profession dismissed the Pritikin experience as anecdotal. But Nathan Pritikin was more of a scientist than most of his critics and he produced proven results that the cholesterol count of those who followed this regimen dropped considerably—sometimes as much as 25% within two to four weeks.

Since then, those who scoffed have adopted much of what Pritikin advocated. The American Heart Association and the American Cancer Society were but two of those who suddenly switched to advocate "Eat less fat."

It is of course possible, as I have demonstrated, that some of the foods approved by the Pritikin approach could be your personal allergies. However one must first accept the premise that your body responds to what you eat and then pursue it from there.

### Eczema

Eczema is another serious and rather vexing ailment.

The medical treatment of eczema includes the use of x-ray, ultraviolet ray, ointments and injection of various vaccines.

Mr. P's physician, after a two months' unrewarded trial of medical treatment of his tormenting eczema, advised him to take the pulse-survey. The pulse reacted to cereals, orange, honey, fowl, lamb, a popular shaving cream (pulse up to 108) and soap powder; and the itch increased markedly soon after he had eaten or used some of these. Three weeks after the elimination of these allergens he was practically well, and for good measure his somewhat elevated blood pressure (140/84) had become normal (about 120/70). At a subsequent visit to his physician something like the following conversation took place:

Doctor: "How are you?"

Mr. P.: "I'm well."

Doctor: "Did Dr. Coca use rays?"

Mr. P.: "No."

Doctor: "Did he give you injections, or something to put on or to take?"

Mr. P.: "No."

Doctor: "Unbelievable!"

Mr. K. was not only covered with an itching and unsightly scaly eruption of several years' duration; he was also about 25 pounds under normal weight, and his blood pressure was disturbingly high, 180/108 in August, and 176/100 in October.

Hearing from a neighbor about the new allergy test which had relieved the neighbor's high blood pressure, he obtained a three-week leave of absence to have the survey made. At the first interview he announced that he was spending the first three days at a beach resort to quiet his mind, and get some "good fresh air." I wished him a pleasant trip, but I assured him that he would be wasting valuable time, and that he was probably not in a frame of mind to benefit from the survey; in blunt fact I did not wish to see him again.

By the next evening I had forgotten about him when he telephoned. I expressed astonishment; he replied, "I fooled you and stayed home counting pulses."

In three weeks' time we had identified egg, fowl, fish, pork, beef, lamb, potato, corn, onions, asparagus and coffee as pulse-accelerating allergens, which were then excluded from his diet.

By the fourth week on the greatly restricted diet he had gained 8 pounds in weight, and the eczema had healed or the body, face, ears, legs and one arm, still persisting on the other forearm and one ankle.

By six weeks the eruption was entirely healed, he had gained 12 pounds, and his company physician reported a nearly normal blood-pressure of 128/78. Three months later he reported dejectedly that "the mess" was back again.

It was almost as bad as ever, and his blood pressure was up (160/84). At first he asserted that he had stuck to his "diet," but after a mild third degree he confessed some indulgence in wine without a pulse-test. I jokingly told him that he could "jump in the lake" and hung up.

After another three weeks I called him. "How are you now?" I asked.

"Oh, I'm well again, it *was* the wine," he replied. His pressure too had returned to normal.

It amazes one to consider that a man of 54 can avoid all the protein-rich meats, also egg and potato, can do harder physical work than ever, yet gain back, as he now has, that 25 pounds of lost weight. That is, he is up to his normal, according to the Thomas D. Wood standard.

## Ulcer

Now look at the "treatment" of ulcer of the stomach. Why, by the way, has no one thought of the similarity of that condition to ulcer of the mouth (the canker sore), which is already recognized as allergic!

First the sufferer usually receives a bland diet such as milk, gelatin, junket; he is given antacids and sedatives; then he is briefed about his anatomy and the "nervous factors." Finally, if all simpler measures fail, surgery is the only apparent solution, and he must submit to an operation known as gastric resection (removal of the ulcer and surrounding parts of the stomach).

This may or may not bring relief to the sufferer. Certainly it seldom cures the underlying cause.

I had not run across my old friend, the chemist, Dr. P. for months when he stopped me and casually remarked that he had an ulcer.

"My dear fellow," I exclaimed, "why the secrecy? Maybe I can help; what are you doing?"

"Well," he replied, "my surgeon is feeding me only milk, and if that doesn't help me he intends soon to operate; and, in fact, I am ready for it because I am worse than ever."

I counted his pulse—104. He found 103. "You have eaten nothing but milk today?" I asked. "Nothing else." "Will you believe in me and do what I say for one week?"

"Yes, but what shall I do?" he asked.

I explained that since he had taken only milk and was running a fast pulse, he was probably allergic to milk. What effect this allergy had on his ulcer remained to be seen. I suggested that he count his pulse before and after meals, eating anything at first *except* milk.

He was skeptical but agreed to give it a try.

At lunch he had a liberal assortment of dishes containing no milk, and his pulse thereafter ranged only from 74 to 78. The result was the same at dinner and at breakfast the following morning, by which time his ulcer-pain had vanished.

Three days in succession this trained scientist tortured himself with a glass of milk at lunch before he was convinced that he could always produce both the pain and the pulse-rise with that food, and that alone—a lucky man!

Another case tells a similar story, but the patient in this instance was not so fortunate. Mr. C. learned about the new test too late to save himself from the gastric resection. Also he learned too late that the operation, if it did not worsen his state, at least did not better it. In fact, six months later he had developed a severe gastritis (inflammation of the stomach-lining) which his physicians had previously assured him was a most unlikely occurrence. A year later, at the age of 46, he was making arrangements to retire from his successfully developed business, physically debilitated to the point where he felt he must take to his bed.

It was from his wife, one of my former laboratory associates, that he heard about the new test, and as a last resort, and with her encouragement he devoted himself conscientiously to the routine counts.

Incidentally, previous routine skin-tests had revealed no allergens. Like Dr. P., he too discovered cow's milk to be his major food-allergen. Moreover, the simple avoidance of cow's milk not only set his sick stomach in peaceful working condition after twenty years of pain and discomfort; but unexpectedly it solved another painful disorder, his hemorrhoids.

Mr. C. is restored to health, to an eight hour day of laborious occupation, and to a serene view of the future in which retirement is too far off to be thought about.


## Hemorrhoids

Hemorrhoids are usually treated at first with neglect, and even their bodily protrusion is viewed only with annoyance so long as they do not become too painful or bleed too freely.

The doctor can recommend only symptomatic relief induced with suppositories, postponing as long as possible the inevitable resort to surgery.

It is remarkable how many of these allergic conditions of previously unknown cause have been "treated" literally according to the biblical counsel, "If thine eye offend thee pluck it out." But here again surgery often fails, just as it does with the different yet comparable instances of adenoids and probably also enlarged tonsils, which also may be the result of allergy.

When the allergic swelling of the nasal mucous membrane extends into the sinuses we call the condition sinusitis. When it involves the membrane covering the ceiling of the posterior cavity of the mouth, the swollen membrane may be thrown into pendulous folds called adenoids. The difference between these and hemorrhoids is that in adenoids there are no swollen veins such as characterize the hemorrhoidal mass. They are similar in that they are both allergic swellings, and that the removal of the presently existing ones does not prevent the formation of others.

Mr. C. had undergone surgery because of painful, bleeding hemorrhoids that protruded. The first operation failed, and a second was advised. Later there occurred an alarming protrusion of a part of the rectum. Even if one admits its possibly food-allergic origin, a dislocation such as this rectal protrusion would not be widely thought reducible through the regulation of the diet. Yet, that's exactly what happened.

It was at this juncture that Mr. C. discovered milk as his sole disturbing food-allergen, and began to exclude it from his diet.

Subsequently improvement was marked and progressive until protrusion had become negligible. Neither had there remained any further bleeding or discomfort.

Mr. M's case was much less serious than that just recounted, but it is illuminating in that after the condition had been miraculously cleared up by mere avoidance of the allergens pea, bean, peanut and tobacco, it returned promptly when bean, unknown to him, was slipped into his diet. It was his migraine headaches and his nagging tired feeling, not his hemorrhoid, that brought him to the pulse-survey.

He did not mention the hemorrhoid until, together with his major complaints, it departed. Indeed several weeks passed before he was sure that it was gone for good, and then its possible connection with his allergy struck him. This result of the new procedure seemed to impress him more than his relief from the other symptoms; it impressed me also, for at that time I had made only one other similar observation.

Mr. M's hemorrhoid did not bleed or protrude, but the pain and discomfort spoiled his night's rest, necessitating the regular use of a suppository. His physician did not wish to risk operation.

In the summer following the disappearance of the condition, Mr. M. took a vacation in good spirits with his restored health. Soon after his arrival at the resort he was disheartened by the recurrence of the hemorrhoidal discomfort.

But the set back was only temporary, because the cause of the trouble was discovered in the soybean and its oil which made its unsuspected way into his diet.

Recently his physician examined him and reported that the hemorrhoid had completely disappeared.

Hemorrhoid by its mass gives the impression of a growth. Yet it is not a growth but a swelling composed largely of distended veins (the conveniently named hemorrhoidal veins).

Now the remarkable disappearance of such a mass following the mere avoidance of pulse-speeding foods spells allergy; and that word is underscored by the prompt recurrence of the mass when one of those foods is unwittingly restored to the diet.

But how explain such a swelling as allergic? This is easily done with the use of common analogies in this amazing field. Let's see.

Young Farmer Jones, against his better judgment based on experience, indulges in some of the first picking from his strawberry patch.

"They won't hurt you," assures his new bride. Next morning Mrs. Jones is wakened by a groan.

"What's the matter, Sam?"

"My head is pounding, and I can't see."

And with obvious reason, for his eyelids are so tensely swollen that they cannot be opened. *Allergic fluid impounded under pressure in the tissues.*

The same phenomenon is apparent in hives, in the intensely swollen, impassable nasal membrane of allergic rhinitis, and in the painful internal pressure of the glaucomatous eye (Berens).

So the original cause of the hemorrhoidal swelling is a collection of allergic fluid localized in the hemorrhoidal area *and restrained* there under pressure. It is this pressure which interferes with the outflow of the blood in the veins, causing them to become distended.

When the "food-allergens" are excluded from the diet, the local allergic process is resolved, the allergic fluid is released, the pressure obstructing the venous circulation is thus removed, and the whole mass disappears like a snowball in an April sun.

### Overweight

Of all the problems that beset modern American man and woman, none consumes as much wasted effort, causes as much talk, or generates as much self-scorn as overweight.

If you are overweight, not merely vanity, but your total state of health is at stake.

Overweight, the bane of so many self-conscious women of tidy instincts, is often "treated" medically, either with controlled starvation, or with a dangerous medicament that helps to burn up excessive fat faster than even the obese person can plough it in.

The fat woman is told that she eats too much, especially sweets and fats, or that she is lazy, or more often, both. But medical science has found a fairer judgment, and a pleasanter way of relief for many such women.

There is now convincing evidence that many cases of overweight are due to food-allergy, and that when the food-allergens are withdrawn from the diet the weight falls to the normal level for the individual, and remains there without any restriction of the safe foods, including starches, sugars and fats.

Little Miss M., age 50, found her physical activity uncomfortably limited by her moderate overweight of nearly 140 pounds. But her daily struggle to negotiate the three flights of steps to her apartment was not due alone to those excessive pounds.

She suffered migraine (climaxed with vomiting), marked tiredness, constipation, occasional dizziness, sinusitis, and, strangely, split finger-nails; which she did not mention until, after the pulse survey was completed, they had rapidly healed.

Cow's milk was her worst allergen, but the others included cereals, all meats but pork (she can eat egg and also goat's milk), citrus fruit and cane sugar.

In the first week of avoidance of these allergens all symptoms disappeared, and she lost four and one-half pounds weight (probably water of allergic edema).

Gradually, in the next four weeks, there was a further loss of three pounds, and ultimately her weight became stable at 129-1/2 pounds.

One's first thought will be starvation (no cereals, no sugar). But there was not any starvation; Miss M. never felt hungry, as she often had when she was fat. She ate to her appetite's content of her many safe foods including potato, sweet potato, dates, peas, beans and (notice this, reader) beet sugar, which she could and did eat freely because she was not allergic to beet.

So Miss M. is proud of her health and her young figure. These three flights of stairs are to her merely a welcome means of exercise, and her advancing age holds no fears for her, because she knows that she has found the key to the prevention of its chief infirmities.

Several other younger women have found the relief of their annoying overweight in the avoidance of their pulse-speeding food-allergens. These, like Miss M., turned to the new procedure primarily on account of more urgent ailments, such as eczema of the hands, migraine and neuralgia. Their return to normal weight was merely an extra dividend happily incidental to the disappearance of the other major and minor allergic symptoms.

Even older women may be grateful beneficiaries of the reducing effects of the nonallergic diet. Two such cases are instructive because the foods that they had to shun were not the fat-producing foods.

These women were over 70 years of age. Both were victims of tiredness and long-standing constipation. Other symptoms in Mrs. P. were heart attacks, fainting, chronic cough and chronic outbreaks of hives ("dollar-size"); in Mrs. B. there was indigestion and migratory neuralgia, with annual six-week bouts with common cold.

After the successful pulse-survey Mrs. P. was free from all listed symptoms, and there was a 15 pound reduction of her weight to a constant normal level.

The quantity of her diet has since been regulated only by her appetite. The food-allergens that she must avoid are beef, cow's milk, egg, corn, orange, olive, banana and yeast. She eats all other cereals, potato and sugar without restriction.

Mrs. B's food-allergens are cow's milk, citrus fruits, carrot, beet, spinach, asparagus, onion and nuts.

Again, no ban against the "fattening" starches and sweets! And *no restriction in quantity*. Yet this woman lost 35 pounds of excessive weight to the great betterment of her well-being and physical activity; not to mention the total recovery from her psychic depression, as well as all her other symptoms. This was fifteen years ago, since which time there have been only occasional dietary lapses, which have quickly brought their own punishment.

Overweight is thought by some medical scientists to predispose to such serious conditions as heart attacks (*angina pectoris*), high blood pressure and diabetes. But now we see that such a theory amounts to charging one symptom of allergy against another.

Overweight does not *cause* hypertension; these two allergic conditions simply are often associated in the same allergic person, and the pulse-dietary survey stands a worthwhile chance to dispel the fraternal ailments together.

A disheartening pronouncement for women of excessive girth comes from the archives of psychiatry. They are told that overweight is a manifestation of a personality disturbance; a neurosis to be "treated" according to psychiatric procedure. Thus another allergic condition is being added to the list of "psychsomatic disorders."

If you are a fat man or a fat woman who may be tempted to consider that proposition, I strongly urge *caveat emptor*; first try counting off the pounds with your finger tips. Discover what thing or things are causing your body to retain the extra weight. Avoid them. And watch the pounds go by.

## Epilepsy

The medical treatment of epilepsy is a sad chapter in modern medicine. You read of such symptomatic treatments such as regulation of the bowels, "mental hygiene," and depressant or antispasmodic drugs, which lessen the seizures in some, but fog the mind in many others.

Relatives are advised to keep the sufferer at home as long as economically and otherwise possible, and when the breaking point is reached there is left only the hope-abandoned refuge of those institutions where 40,000 others wait either for the mental blackout or for death.

Mr. F. came to me for relief of his headaches, indigestion, stiffening joints and marked abnormal tiredness. He had an epileptic sister, and as a young man he had suffered *grand mal* seizures. But he was not aware of the numerous brief *petit mal* episodes which had been observed in him by his wife in the past 20 years. His major food-allergen is orange.

About a month after he had stopped eating orange, his wife told me for the first time about the epilepsy, and stated that the seizures had ceased. He has remained free thereafter, and all of his other symptoms departed at the same time. Incidentally, he lost 25 pounds of his overweight.

The next four cases came to me in the following year. These are described elsewhere in this book. The dramatic outcome in one of them (B.B.) is touchingly conveyed in the letter from his nurse to my friend S.

Dear S.:

But I have wonderful news to report. B. B. is cured under Dr. Coca's treatment. It seems like a miracle, but he really acts like another person. He had a "mumbling" of speech at times, and it was difficult to understand him. That has disappeared entirely, and he speaks very distinctly.

He gets up in the morning happy and singing with a clear mind. He says he used to get up feeling confused. The other night he said he entered into a debate and found he could think very quickly and clearly, which he could not do before. It was hard to think quickly.

He also played football the other day—he hasn't done this for years—and felt no ill effects—he says he is "as happy as a lark," and I am equally happy as I love the boy very much.

He is a fine person; but he was doomed—and now he is . well. It seems too wonderful to believe.

K.R. (nurse)

Note from "S":

"This epileptic boy has had a rather wide experience, having had brain-wave charts, etc. made, with many experts in New York and Boston before this food-allergy idea was tried."

Eight epileptic persons have been given this full anti-allergic "treatment," five having had the conservative sympathectomy, and these eight have satisfactorily observed the indicated restrictions. One of these, a "mentally retarded" boy of seven, after a year's daily consultations must be counted at present a failure.* In six the seizures are prevented by avoidance of the identified allergens, and they are controlled in the seventh by a small daily dose of dilantin, which was not tolerated previous to the sympathectomy.

Epileptic seizures can be prevented in the large majority of cases. But by far the more important conclusion from these experiences is that the cause of that dreadful affliction has at last been brought to light. It is "food-allergy."

---

*The failure of the pulse-dietary procedure in this case found explanation or parallel in the complete failure of the method in all of 14 cases of epilepsy that were thoroughly studied in Rockland State Hospital, N.Y. All of the 14 were also afflicted with a psychosis. The pulse-dietary method failed also in 6 other patients in the same institution who were subjects of dementia praecox and not epileptic. The damage caused by the psychotic localization in the brain thus appears to be irreversible. Such a condition, then, may be preventable but not curable.

## Hives

Hives, the plain English word for urticaria, is one of the most widely known allergic conditions. Its medical treatment, as described in some standard text-books, reveals the general lack of knowledge of its cause.

Among the listed excitants of hives we do find foods mentioned, but only *certain* foods. One author warns especially against shellfish, strawberries, mushrooms, pork, nuts and, less urgently, cereals. Neither will he allow his patients to eat egg, "meats except lamb and poultry" (why these exceptions?), tomato, sweets, jellies, alcohol, tea or coffee. But such a list represents only a hit-or-miss shot-gun selection.

Incidentally, his list of possible excitants includes table-salt (sodium chloride), which cannot cause any kind of allergy.

The books approve grandmother's castor oil treatment. They also offer vaccines, "alkaline diet," bicarbonate of soda and various drugs. But the most remarkable measure is the withdrawal of blood from the vein of the patient, and injection of it into his buttock. (And strangely this sometimes helps!)

One author concludes that the medical treatment is purely symptomatic and unscientific, and that every effort should be made to determine the cause.

Well, the pulse-method is the tool with which the cause or causes of hives *can* now be discovered, and the results of its use have been gratifying and sometimes astonishing.

Mrs. P., age 70, was the first sufferer from hives (dollar-size) to make her escape from this misery through the pulse-counts. The pulse-speeding foods, all of which, one after the other, caused outbreaks of hives were beef, orange, banana, egg, olive, corn and yeast.

It is a mysterious fact that not all of an allergic person's food-allergens cause hives. J. C.'s allergens are wheat, sugar and coffee; but his hives were caused only by coffee. Wheat and sugar caused only migraine and indigestion. C. G.'s allergens are wheat and beef, but only wheat causes hives.

Foods are not the only excitants of hives. A. McC.'s rest was ruined night after night by outbreaks of huge itching welts. It is noted elsewhere in this book that as soon as dust-proof coverings were applied to her bedding the nocturnal attacks ceased.

## Food-allergens

Long ago, the allergist Warren T. Vaughan reported that most allergic people blame their digestive troubles on the onion and cabbage. If his patient was allergic to egg the meal would "repeat" as he called it; but it was not the egg he tasted in that event, it was the harmless onion or cabbage he had eaten with it.

Now when we look through the records of 100 food-allergic patients and list the foods to which each was found allergic with the use of the pulse reaction, we find that the most frequent excitants of the food allergies are just the commonly eaten foods. This is indicated in the table on the next page.

Since these figures tell the number of affected persons among 100 tested, and since about 90 percent of the population are victims of food-allergy, the figures represent

| Food | Number of persons allergic to it | Food | Number of persons allergic to it | Food | Number of persons allergic to it |
|---|---|---|---|---|---|
| egg | 33 | tomato | 19 | fowl | 15 |
| wheat | 30 | banana | 19 | melon | 14 |
| white potato | 30 | onion | 19 | carrot | 13 |
| cow's milk | 29 | asparagus | 19 | sw. potato | 13 |
| orange | 29 | cabbage | 18 | grape | 12 |
| beef | 23 | pork | 18 | peanut | 12 |
| pea, bean | 22 | chocolate | 17 | pineapple | 12 |
| fish | 20 | lamb | 17 | beet, spinach | 11 |
| sugar cane | 20 | coffee | 15 | corn | 10 |
| plum | 21 | apple | 15 | yeast | 9 |
|  |  |  |  | strawberry | 6 |

approximately the percentage of the population who are allergic to the respective food. For example, about 30 percent of the people are allergic to egg, and over 25 percent to wheat, potato, milk and orange.

The most acute allergic misery can be caused by very small quantities of some of these foods. One extremely egg-sensitive man could detect the egg in a dilution of 1 to 50,000 when a drop of it was placed on his tongue. Even this weak solution caused an instant burning sensation, and his reaction always warned him in time to prevent him from swallowing food mixtures containing egg, at the risk of a dangerous allergic shock.

Asthmatic attacks have been caused by the mere fumes from frying bacon or buckwheat cakes, even when the cooking was going on in a neighboring apartment.

One sensitive to sugar cane suffered his dizziness after swallowing less than one-tenth millionth of a milligram of the cane protein.

Purity in the matter of food means one thing to the officials of the Food and Drug Administration, but something remarkably different to allergy-torn humanity. The federal authorities used to permit food-packers to list "vegetable oil" on their labels. So the purchaser who happened to be exquisitely allergic to soy-bean had to learn the hard way that his food package contains his particular poison—soy-bean oil.

The government-approved term "vegetable shortening" is also a pitfall for allergic people. Sugar is sugar to the administration, but not to the occasional harassed victim of allergy caused by beet-sugar.

(Editor's note: The FDA has, in recent years, improved the information required on food labels.)

Patient A. had long enjoyed his strawberries "frozen in sugar." They were his only tolerated fruit. One day his customary brand went off the market, and very soon thereafter he suffered a severe and continuing recurrence of one of his most fearsome allergic symptoms—intestinal hemorrhage. The earlier attacks of hemorrhage had been proved to be allergic, but this one had to be of a different cause since, *so far as he knew,* his diet had not changed.

His wife solved the mystery; first by recalling the change in the package of berries, and then by finding out that the new brand was packed most probably in the Middle West with beet-sugar. The patient is allergic to beet.

The neighbors took over the rest of the frozen stock, and patient A. turned safely to fresh strawberries with cane sugar, to which he is not allergic.

You are probably familiar with many of these foods superstitions:

People with "weak digestion" are warned against *fried* food, hard boiled egg, too fresh bread, pork, cheese, coffee and other good things. Boiled milk is said to be constipating, and prunes laxative; ice-cream according to one superstition should not be eaten with shellfish. Some would eat only soft foods, while others add bran and other roughage to the diet as stimulants of bowel activity.

All of these ideas arise from experiences with the food-allergic stomach and intestine. The fried-food phobia comes from an observer who could eat the boiled or roasted food with impunity, but not the same food if it was fried in a fat to which he was allergic. Mr. F. accused the diner cook of poisoning the sausages, which at home he ate without getting cramps in his stomach. But his allergy-wise dining companion drew from the cook the fact that his sausages were fried in perfectly pure Crisco, to which he, among a few other people, happens to be allergic.

Your *non-allergic* stomach digests the fried foods as well as the boiled or broiled. If you are allergic to prunes they may cause diarrhea *for you;* then they are laxative.

Hard-boiled egg if normally chewed is easily digested, each particle becoming surrounded with a film of the digestive juice.

That burning sensation of the stomach known as "heartburn" may not be due to hyperacidity, but to the allergic irritation of the lining membrane. Tobacco smoke causes it in some tobacco-allergic persons even when the stomach is practically empty; and then it may sometimes be first noticed after swallowing just a little pure water.

"Bolting one's food" is universally condemned. You

don't need to read the Russian scientist Pavlov to believe that the digestive apparatus is healthfully stimulated by the more prolonged influence of the aromas, and the flavors of appetizing food, as well as by the more thorough chewing of it. However, the *non-allergic* stomach and other digestive organs are able and willing to manage even bolted food without symptomatic resentment.

The point is that you should not try to humor your allergically sick insides with "easily digestible, non-irritating soft diets."

The secret of improved health and happier living rests in this simple formula; stop abusing yourself with *your* particular food-poisons and other allergens.

You'll be pleased with the results.

Note that since this book was originally written, the approach advocated by Nathan Pritikin and described earlier, has changed the way Americans think about the foods they eat.

For example, I talked about eggs but Pritikin advocates only egg whites. He is a strong opponent of any diet which includes ingesting more than a few ounces of animal protein a day. As his cause has triumphed, fewer Americans eat beef on a regular basis. The consumption of eggs, butter, bacon, and red meat, has fallen.

# (7)

# High Blood Pressure?

The layman may be excused if he blames his high blood pressure on some misbehavior of his arteries. But medical science has discovered a substance "angiotonin" which is liberated from the *kidney*, and is believed to cause a tightening of the arteries that results in the increase of pressure on the circulating blood.

This can very well be true but, as you will now see, the *primary cause of the liberation of angiotonin which had eluded detection is "food-allergy" affecting the kidney.*

The circulation of the blood takes place within a closed elastic-walled system composed of the heart and the blood vessels. The blood fills the system to the point of slight stretching of its walls, whereby the fluid is constantly under a pressure.

The so-called diastolic pressure is that which exists *between* the heart-beats. It was said by the physiologist, William H. Howell, to equal the pressure of a column of mercury 65 to 75 millimeters high, in the normal man. The contraction of the heart puts a momentary additional "pulse pressure" on the system, which increases the basic diastolic pressure up to 110 to 116 millimeters of mercury. This is called the systolic pressure.

These two pressures are those found in the heavy-coated arteries. The pressure in the more thinly walled vein is usually unaffected by the pulse, and is much lower.

The blood pressures recorded in medical practice are those of the arteries in the upper arm, and taking as an example the figures of Dr. Howell, they are noted like this—116/75.

The figures of Dr. Howell are surely within the normal range, yet the limits of that range have not been determined. The reason for this is that abnormally high blood-pressure is found in so large a proportion of adults, and even in some children.

Thus there have been no standards against which to judge whether a systolic pressure of 140 may actually represent the maximal figure of the normal range as some assume, or is a truly abnormal pressure. That is, whether it is always evidence of early hypertension.

It is not important to the individual's immediate health to decide whether a systolic pressure of 140 means the beginning of hypertension or not; because that and even considerably higher pressures can be tolerated indefinitely in almost all persons without the slightest risk. Nevertheless, the allergic patient with a pressure of 140 who is seeking relief from his itching eczema and migraine is agreeably impressed to see that pressure drop to 120 or even lower as his other symptoms disappear after he has eliminated his food-allergens from his diet.

Once again I must credit the Nathan Pritikin approach

to diet with very effective control of blood pressure. This has not proved to be the all-encompassing answer but the simple switch to a diet consisting largely of vegetables, complex carbohydrates, beans, etc., combined with exercise four to six days a week (this can be as simple as walking a couple of miles a day or spending forty minutes a day on a treadmill) has, with certainty, reduced blood pressure in thousands of cases.

"Average" blood pressures have been determined by numerous physicians in large groups of individuals; but no practical use for such averages has come from those studies. This is because hypertension was found in all groups in all circumstances of age, sex and season. And even opinion concerning the significance of pressures greater than 140 in student groups was evaded with the remark "only time will tell what it is." Well, time has now caught up with the question, and the answer is in your pulse rate.

The idea that high blood pressure can be a consequence of "food-allergy" did not come to me out of the blue. It did not come as a "hunch" which I proceeded to investigate. It arrived as a kind of *fait accompli* out of routine examinations of the blood pressure before and in the period of the dietary treatment of allergic symptoms in two patients.

The first readings were not big enough (136, 140) to rate as indications of hypertension; but the pressure in the first case was distinctly higher than it had been on all the many occasions of earlier examination in that individual through his adult life of about 40 years.

That fact stirred his curiosity, but only faintly, until after the exclusion of all his food-allergens of the moment the pressure dropped about 20 points, and remained there. When the same sequence occurred in the second patient the idea was born, and the chase for proof was on.

These two cases might be significant, but more definite proof was required.

First, the pulse-dietary procedure had to be applied in an undoubted case of hypertension; that is, one of sufficient duration, in an elderly person with a blood-pressure greater than 150/90.

I found such a case in Mrs. E. A., 60 years of age. Her physicians for some time had warned her of her high pressure, which sometimes reached 198/120. Sixteen days after avoidance of her major food-allergens the pressure was 112/78.

Second, resumption of the eating of the food-allergens must be followed by a rise in the pressure. This happened also in the case of Mrs. E. A. who abandoned her dietary restrictions on the 23rd day. On the 26th day the pressure was 138/104. Return to her restrictions was again followed by a fall of the pressure, which gradually arrived at 114/74. Then she began eating one of her allergens, wheat, and again the pressure gradually increased to 142/84.

She finally decided to be "good." She stopped eating wheat, and in the next month the pressure sank gradually to 124/72.

Third, the relief of the hypertension that follows the anti-allergic regime must hold as long as the treatment continues, and for at least three to five years. The treatment of Mrs. E. A. began decades ago, and in spite of the steadily increasing demands on her energies in the making of fine candies, she feels and looks better than ever, and her pressure remains in the lower range, subject only to occasional minor lapses in her restrictions.

The latest figures taken are still 124/70.

Fourth, the treatment must be regularly effective depending on the identification of *all* the allergens. This requirement was met in six other cases. It was not met in the two persons in whom the allergens were not all identified.

Fifth and finally, the proof which was gathered in the foregoing experiences had still to be tested by other competent unprejudiced observers. This also has been done. At first independently, by Dr. A. Sumner Price, whose report appeared in the *Review of Gastroenterology*, and later by Dr. Milo G. Meyer, reporting before the New York Academy of Sciences.

How can allergy cause hypertension?

For one-half of the answer to this question we turn to the classical experiments of Dr. H. Goldblatt, which have been solidly confirmed. With the use of a specially designed small metal clamp Dr. Goldblatt compressed the artery supplying the kidney of the dog so that the flow of blood through the organ was not stopped but only slowed. The clamp was left in place for the remainder of the period of observation.

If the flow was moderately retarded, the animal's blood-pressure was moderately increased. If the flow was still further retarded the blood-pressure rose still further, and there followed arteriosclerosis (hardening of the arteries) in different parts of the body, which is seen so regularly in the late stages of human hypertension.

Hypertension could also be produced in the dog if the blood current was slowed by compression of the kidney itself with a sac placed about the organ.

Now this promising line of research ended temporarily in a blind alley because laboratory scientists could not imagine any natural, physiological cause of the compression of all the blood-vessels of both kidneys in the hypertensive human being to compare with the Goldblatt experiment. Yet such a cause is not hard to imagine in terms of allergy. Let us examine this.

The "hive" is a typical allergic manifestation, and certainly it is one that is familiar to many of us. The most important feature of the hive is not the itching nor the red flare that often forms its periphery; it is the *tense, pale,* swelling at the center. The tenseness and pallor are the effects of *internal pressure* caused by the collection of allergic edematous fluid which is hindered from normal escape by some allergic obstruction. It is worth while to examine this fundamental phenomenon more closely.

Your normal body tissues are being constantly flushed with a fluid known as lymph. The lymph is really derived from the blood, being filtered through the walls of your smallest blood vessels by the force of the blood pressure. The fluid has not the slightest red color since the pores through which it is filtered are too minute for the escape of the red blood cells.

Outside the blood vessels the lymph is normally pushed into the openings of another system of narrow channels known as lymph vessels. These vessels join with others of their kind. The system finally empties into one of the large veins.

One important injurious effect of the allergic reaction is a local blockade of the lymph vessels.

How this is brought about is not known; but its effect is obvious. As more fluid is filtered into the allergically involved area under the force of the blood pressure, the pressure in the area finally becomes so great that no further filtration is possible. This collection of lymph under restraint and internal pressure is now called "edema."

When in such a situation all the allergens are avoided, the reaction passes, the allergic obstruction yields, the fluid gradually escapes, and normal conditions are restored with usually no lasting damage to the area.

This important feature of internal pressure characterizes a number of the visually accessible manifestations of allergy (nasal, asthmatic, ocular—glaucoma—meningeal, as in migraine). Hence it is reasonable to surmise that allergy, which has been proved to be at least a common cause of human hypertension, produces that condition through the *internal pressure* of allergic edema affecting both kidneys.

This pressure slows the flow of blood through these organs, and so establishes the conditions of the Goldblatt experiment.

# (8)

## "Tobacco Poisoning"

Since the time of that famous quarrel between pope Urban VIII and James I over tobacco-smoking, Lady Nicotine has been a subject of controversy, if the feeble struggle of her detractors against the overwhelming numbers of her devotees can be so named.

The habitual smoker offends many a non-smoker. This objection is reflected in the growing number of "no smoking" signs in public places. But recent scientific study has revealed a much more serious indictment of the American weed. Tobacco turns out to be a powerful allergen affecting more than three-fourths of the population.

The damaging effects of smoking are presently being brought to public attention in front-page sensational reports by investigators and by-line "science-writers." They all seem to be wholly unacquainted with the *nature* of those damaging effects, though this has been reported in the past by myself and by Dr. Granville F. Knight, of

Santa Barbara, California. Dr. Knight is past President of the American Academy of Nutrition.

A statistical survey covering 187,766 men between the ages of 25 and 70 has shown that the death rate of the smokers in that group was 75 percent higher than that of non-smokers.

Had that survey been conducted by persons acquainted with the fundamental principles concerning the new allergy, it would have been discovered: 1) that between 8,000 and 10,000 of the whole group were, by inheritance, not allergic: 2) that none of these had suffered either heart-attacks or cancer: 3) that the death rate in this nonallergic group was relatively very low, the deaths being due largely to accident or infection: and 4) that smoking had no deleterious effect on any of the nonallergic group.

Heart damage and cancer are but two of the more common dividends paid by cigarettes to their smokers.

In February 1982, the Surgeon General of the United States, Dr. C. Everett Koop, broadened the list of cancers linked to cigarettes. He charged that in addition to lung cancer, cigarette smoking has clearly been linked to bladder, kidney and pancreatic cancers. It has also been linked to stomach cancer and uterine cervical cancer.

Dr. Koop declared that 30 percent of all cancer deaths are attributable to smoking.

Many smokers are hard people to convince. If you were handed a knife and I told you to cut your wrist a little each day, or to dig its point into your stomach a quarter of an inch each week, you would shudder and back away from me.

Yet, if you are a confirmed smoker, you may be doing more severe and lasting damage to yourself.

Not all people are allergic to cigarettes, of course. But so many are that you owe it to yourself to test yourself.

This is what one experiment with cigarettes revealed during pulse dietary surveys. Thirty-eight "food-allergic" persons counted their pulse before and after they began the test, usually by smoking a cigarette.

Nineteen showed no significant change in their pulse count, although some continued smoking for periods of fifteen minutes to one hour.

The other 19 recorded increased rates occurring within a few minutes, usually 3 to 6 minutes, and sometimes even as soon as one minute.

One man's rate increased from 85 to 119 within 6 minutes, and the rate of one 11-year-old boy who had merely held a cold tobacco-pipe in his mouth, increased from 84 to 104 in 9 minutes.

The allergic symptoms caused by tobacco are just as various as are those caused by any food-allergen.

A prominent chemical investigator who was collaborating with me upon the question of body-odors begged me to rescue him from his continual headaches, tiredness, and "nervous indigestion." He also suffered from frequently recurring neuralgia.

I advised him to make a preliminary survey of the pulse on his usual diet before undertaking the systematic tests of single foods. During this period he reluctantly agreed not to smoke.

At the end of one week he and his wife visited me, both in a state of joyful excitement; he was completely free from all his symptoms, and restored to exuberant health and physical activity.

Through the week on his regular varied diet his pulse had remained between 68 and 78, a normal range. There were no food-allergens. However, his curiosity plus the habitual urge had led him on several evenings to make a test of a single cigarette. Each time his pulse ran far above its normal range, reaching 90 to 92. This effect wore off in the night.

The case seemed to be happily solved; but I was wrong. Sometime later he gave me an evasive answer to my inquiry about his health. When I pressed him he confessed that he had resumed smoking, that since he now knew the cause of his symptoms they did not worry him. Besides, he alibied, he could practice "moderation" whenever they bit too deeply.

There has been a more gratifying outcome in the case of attractive 28-year-old Mrs. S., who had long suffered from "deadly tiredness," nervousness, fearfulness, constant "chest colds," painful, crampy menstruation and constipation.

In the first two days of the test her pulse-counts ranged from 60 to 104, with no extraordinary exertion. From that time she was advised to stop smoking, after which the pulse gradually slowed to a maximum of 74 and a minimum of 70.

No pulse-accelerating foods were discovered, but two tests with cigarette-smoking resulted in a rise of the pulse count within five minutes to 98 and 100 respectively.

After six weeks of avoiding tobacco, she reported "feeling marvelous, unbelievable, no aches, that tired feeling gone, no morning mucus, no fears, sleep well and a painless period—first ever." The colds had ceased, and there was a gratifying nine-pound gain of weight to 127 pounds (height 5 feet 6-½ inches).

All of the physical and mental afflictions of this young woman including the painful periods had been attributed to "nerves." The modern medical $64,000 label for the lady's condition is "psychoneurosis," but what she yearned for was not its name but its cause. And that is just what she found out with her finger-tips and her watch—in less than six weeks.

A good variety of allergic symptoms have been proved to be caused by tobacco. Some I have mentioned. There are others, one of the most startling of which is epileptic seizure, which has followed exposure to tobacco smoke in three subjects.

In the first, a girl of 11 years, a *petit mal* reaction occurred within a few minutes after she began breathing through the folds of a handkerchief into which cigarette smoke had just been blown.

The second epileptic girl, age 18, had had a limited sympathectomy, which had left only a small list of "food-allergens," chiefly egg. In the following three months she was in daily technical service, and with two exceptions, free from seizures.

On the two occasions while she was avoiding all "food-allergens," she was heavily exposed at her apartment to cigarette and cigar smoke. Each time she suffered a seizure; once without convulsion and once with typical *grand mal* convulsions. On both occasions the seizures occurred very soon, in about a half hour, after the exposure to the smoke.

The third epileptic patient, a man of thirty years, came for help in 1941, in danger of losing his advanced position in a large corporation. His vice-president told me that if I failed the young man was ruined, because he was having seizures in public places, and soon would be forced into an institution.

When I explained to the patient the new method of identifying the causes of the seizures he readily agreed deliberately to induce a "spell" with one of his allergens. This he did eight months later without advance word to me, and he chose for his experiment tobacco, which had caused a pulse rise of 102 in the single test, and which in the meantime, along with his numerous food-allergens, had been strictly avoided.

He began smoking on a Thursday. On waking Saturday he was *gratified* to notice sensations which he recognized as those formerly presaging a seizure. He resumed smoking, and in the mid-afternoon fell in a major convulsive seizure, in which he was attended by a nearby physician.

I can never recall the quiet, purposeful courage marking that lonely act without a misty eye and a grateful heart. Doubtless this will stand in medical history as one of the first experimental productions of allergic epilepsy in man. It is matched only in the case of a younger boy who twice at six-month intervals deliberately induced a major seizure by eating wheat.

The young man has not smoked in the subsequent ten years, and has faithfully observed his rather stringent dietary restrictions. In that period there have been no seizures; and he always assures me, by the way, that his former unpleasant irritability has been replaced by an equable disposition.

Another serious consequence of the allergic effect of tobacco is high blood-pressure and heart attacks. Physicians have long recognized the relationship of smoking to these conditions, yet without ever suspecting its allergic nature. Medical advice to their hypertensive patients is frequently to "smoke less" rather than to abstain completely.

However, the advice to smoke less cannot stand up before the fact that blood-pressure has been greatly increased following mere exposure to the smoke of others.

On one occasion a hypertensive man went for an automobile drive with a cigar-smoker; his previous diastolic blood pressure had been 74 and 78, but an hour and a half after the drive that pressure stood at 96, and after four and a half hours it was 100.

Surprisingly small quantities of tobacco smoke are capable of upsetting its allergic victims in many ways. A smoker's overcoat or even his breath when not smoking may convey cruel and somewhat prolonged distress to his allergic host—heartburn, diarrhea, smarting eyes, and many others.

It is worth bearing in mind that this same consideration applies also to other air-carried allergic excitants. The following shorthand notes taken out of a letter from J. J. O'Neill impresses this fact:

Bill Jones thinks it was the liquor Joe Jinks served last night that knocked his stomach for a loop the next morning, whereas it was the smoke of Hank Hawkins' cigar. John Q. Manager comes home with his nerves on edge, appetite off, and blames it on the strain of his job. It is the dense atmosphere in the smoker during his card game on the 5:15. Bessie Bargain is knocked out after a day of shopping in the city. It wasn't the work she did but the exhaust fumes of the busses.

These unstudied imaginary illustrations strike close to actual occurrences in the allergist's experience.

A nurse exquisitely sensitive to cat hair was unable to visit her mother's home because of the family cat. So the mother made the long trip to see her daughter. Immediately after her arrival the nurse began to suffer an asthmatic attack which lasted three days; that is, until all the mother's clothes had been cleared of the cat dander she had brought with her.

Although many allergic persons have come for the pulse dietary survey for a particular major symptom such as asthma, hypertension, eczema, diabetes, or migraine, the whole symptomatic picture in most of them adds up to one of "psychoneurosis" or "psychosomatic disorder." Only a few of those persons had consulted a psychiatrist, but the story of one of those who had done so is of startling significance. I call it the case of dad's tobacco-pipe.

G. F., a highly intelligent, beautiful brunette of 24 years, ordinarily of a cheerful, friendly nature became moody, melancholic, extremely irritable, and given to hysterical weeping spells. She was afflicted also with hives, canker sores, abdominal pain and diarrhea.

In complete discourgement she gave up her position, staying at home under her doctor's orders. X-ray examination showed nothing abnormal, but that favorable information only depressed her because she knew that something *was very wrong* with her health, and the X-ray had merely failed to show what it was.

She tried the doctor's prescription hopefully for a while, but lost four pounds in a few weeks, reaching a low of 94 pounds (with a height of 5 feet and 1 ¾ inches). Then she refused medication.

Finally a psychiatrist was called in, mainly to persuade the girl to take her medicines. He made a valiant but vain effort.

On one occasion as she was sitting quietly by a table reading, she suddenly experienced a violent hysterical attack that seemed to come upon her out of the blue. As she rose from her chair she noticed a visitor's half-burned cigar on an ash-tray by her elbow, but no thought of its allergic significance occurred to her till later when she took the tobacco test. Her father is a constant pipe-smoker.

At long last she was enticed into the home of relatives who do not smoke, and who persuaded her against her skepticism to take the pulse-survey. On the third day, having found nothing in a varied diet that disturbed her pulse, she tested tobacco (cigarette). As she began to smoke the count was 72; in three minutes it stood at 92, and she stopped smoking.

When this result was reported to her father he immediately got rid of his smoking outfit, and forbade anyone else to smoke in the house. On the fourth day G.F. went home, and on the eighth she reported a gain of two pounds, and "the appetite of a horse." She had found a new position, and was restored in body and spirit, knowing now what had really been the matter with her and how to correct it. G. F.'s jinx did not come from her "nerves" but from dad's tobacco-pipe.

The allergy to tobacco, affecting at least three-fourths of the population, according to a more recent estimate by Dr. Granville F. Knight, must rate as a primary public *health* problem.

Meanwhile, you are becoming one of the "elite" in that you understand the significance of the problem of tobacco, and know that it relates to the overall problem of food allergy.

For the proper performance of the "smoking test," it is necessary, *first*, to establish the normal pulse-range in the individual; secondly, to choose a time for the test when the pulse is within the limits of that normal range. Count the pulse before beginning to smoke and five times at three minute intervals while smoking.

If the pulse does not rise within 15 minutes above its normal maximum, the individual is not allergic to tobacco and will not be harmed by it.

"Sniff-tests" of other inhaled allergens (powders, scrapings, gasoline, perfume) can be similarly made.

It's worth noting that the publisher of this book has practiced what he preaches. Years ago when the *Wall Street Journal* did a survey to find those companies who'd banned cigarette smoking on their premises, the Campbell Soup Company was revealed to have had such a ban in effect for more than one hundred years. The company that had the second-longest such history was Lyle Stuart Inc. Smoking was banned throughout the offices and warehouses for more than thirty years.

# (9)

# The "House Dust" Problem

There are people who are allergic not to any food, but only to a substance they inhale. More, these substances are sometimes harder to avoid than the food-allergens.

We've talked about tobacco. Another substance to which many people are allergic is bedding or upholstery-dust, etc. This has been loosely classified as "house dust," though it is something quite apart from the dust that you breathe in the street, or that which flows into your home through an open window.

The inhaled allergens have been known to cause many of the symptoms also caused by food-allergens. Specifically, I can cite cases of asthma, stuffy nose, headache, neuralgia, arthritis, multiple sclerosis, diarrhea, eczema and hypertension that have resulted from house dust allergy.

There is a product called *Dust-Seal* produced especially to relieve this problem by L. S. Green Associates, at 162 West 56th Street, New York, NY 10019. I have found it to produce excellent results. An inquiry to the manufacturer will bring you particulars.

There are some people who are allergic only to "house dust." There are others to whom a "house dust" allergy is a secondary thing, which only becomes a clear health danger when the food allergens have been discovered and avoided for a time.

You may wonder that I enclose the term "house dust" in quotes. This is because I want to avoid misleading you. I don't want you to assume that "house dust" refers to the myriad bits of household fabrics which swarm the atmosphere of the home, eventually congregating on polished flat surfaces, or drifting into corners or under beds. That this impression is incorrect is indicated by the following:

1. In the first study of the "house dust" allergen the substance was not found (by extraction) in new, unused furnishings.

2. It is specifically the same substance whether it is found in cotton, or wool, or other fabrics.

3. The substance is not found in outdoor dust, and is present in negligible quantity in dust collected with a vacuum in an uncarpeted hall.

4. The "house dust" allergen appears in mattresses and other furnishings *after* they have been in household use.

5. After all the reservoirs of the "house dust" allergen have been locked up with Dust-Seal, dust particles continue to pervade the atmosphere of the home; yet the dust *allergen* is practically absent in those particles.

In consideration of these facts the conclusion was reached that the "house dust" allergen does not represent any physical or chemical product of the fabrics constituting house furnishings; and that the dust-allergen is produced by some unidentified microorganism(s) which grows in the fabrics.

It was in 1948 that the seemingly hopeless battle against the mysterious "dust-allergen" was simply and inexpensively won. Here is the story of the last decisive round.

The closing up of bed mattresses, pillows, cushions, and the stuffing of upholstered furniture with dust-proof covers had brought relief to some dust-sensitive persons. But many other victims, especially asthmatic persons, and those afflicted with high blood pressure still remained in a precarious condition.

The person with high blood pressure still had to seek additional measure of avoidance by living in his enclosed sun-porch, and had to leave the house altogether during the house-cleaning operations. The asthmatic woman suffered attacks of difficult breathing whenever the vacuum cleaner or dust cloth was in use.

It was the friendly, altruistic advice of a representative of a ventilating company that manufactures a well-known filter for home and office protection against hay fever pollens, which led to the use of an air-filter to clear the atmosphere in the house from dust.

As soon as the filter was installed the symptoms were greatly relieved, and mankind was brought a good step nearer the final solution of the dust problem.

The filter was useful, marvelously so in some cases, but it had some drawbacks. It was too expensive for some families. It encroached, inconveniently in some homes on precious space. It was not automatic in operation, and had to be turned on *and* off at different times, depending on the household activities. It fell short, sometimes seriously, of the perfection of the dust-proof covers in holding the dust-allergen at the source of its production.

It seemed likely that the principal remaining source of the atmosphere dust-allergen was the carpets and rugs. But how to seal off these obviously uncoverable dust-reservoirs? By a lucky coincidence the means for the solution of this problem was at hand.

I have referred to a product named Dust-Seal. Dust-Seal consists of a highly diluted milk-white emulsion which is applied to rugs and carpets, etc., etc. It causes no stickiness to the fabric, and leaves no visible trace of its presence.

To the frightened sufferers from high blood pressure or asthma due to dust-sensitivity, the immediate relief following this treatment with Dust-Seal has been truly magical. And there are other benefits. The air-filter is made quite superfluous because the dust-allergen, being immobilized at its source, or perhaps no longer produced there, does not get into the air at all.

In communities that are not troubled with excessive coal-dust or smoke, or other extraneous dusts (which, by the way are ordinarily not excitants of allergy) the routine house-cleaning is perceptibly lightened through the dust-catching property of Dust-Seal.

So, at least, the difficult problem of avoidance of the dust-allergen has been solved with a minimum of expense and inconvenience. This development increases the prospect of the successful use of the pulse-dietary course in the control of both high blood pressure and bronchial asthma, as well as many other allergic symptoms of dust-sensitivity.

The subsequent eight-year experiences with the use of Dust-Seal have revealed unexpected facts relating to dust-sensitivity.

The first observed manifestations of allergy to dust were those affecting the respiratory tract, asthma and the symptoms resembling "hay-fever." In such cases the specific sensitivity to dust could often be confirmed with the familiar skin-tests carried out with extracts of dust that had been collected with a vacuum cleaner.

The discovery of the allergic pulse reaction (acceleration) permitted the recognition of dust-sensitivity in persons in whom the skin-test is "negative."

For example, if the pulse is markedly quickened following a furniture-dusting operation, or after making the beds; or if the pulse-rate is even slightly higher on waking in the morning than on retiring, this can throw strong suspicion upon dust as an allergic trouble maker.

With the use of such criteria a number of instances have been encountered in which "house-dust" was the sole cause of the allergic symptoms, and in some of these cases the symptoms were not respiratory. The following case histories are astonishing examples.

Mr. B., age 74, had suffered through the past ten years from an eczematoid condition which affected his feet and legs so severely that he was unable to wear shoes, and had to change his socks frequently because of the exudation from the swollen and fissured skin.

He was found not to be allergic to any food except the

cabbage family and onion, which he never ate because they caused migraine headache.

Smoking did not affect his pulse, and by these exclusions "house-dust" was left as the only suspect. Bedding and house furnishings were Dust-Sealed, and immediately his pulse-range dropped four points. Within a few weeks the eczematous lesions were healed, and he could wear shoes. There has been no recurrence.

Mr. W., age 32, suddenly began to have daily attacks of painless vomiting. Thorough X-ray and other examinations in two U.S. Marine hospitals revealed no organic abnormalities. It was noticed that the attacks were more frequent (as many as four times) on a Sunday when he remained at home. There were no food sensitivities, and he was not pulse-sensitive to tobacco.

On his first visit to my office Mr. W. brought with him a pulse record covering two days. The "retiring" count one evening was 70, but on waking next morning he found that the rate before getting out of bed was 74.

He was willing to accept this finding as an indication of probably dust-sensitivity, and on the following day he applied Dust-Seal to his bedding and other furniture in his apartment. That night he slept elsewhere and vomited as usual. In the several years since his return to his apartment he has vomited only twice; once after helping his sister move her furniture, and again after staying over night at a relative's apartment.

Mr. X is a sensitive, cultured gentleman, successful in business, his retirement not very distant. His one weakness spoiled his otherwise pleasant outlook; he was a compulsive secret drinker—a victim of "alcoholism."

Mr. X's married daughter, who has been thoroughly indoctrinated in the pulse-dietary procedure, recently told me the following:

"For a number of years my father had been a secret compulsive drinker, although he never drank to the point of visible inebriation. He never drank socially, probably not wishing to appear interested in alcoholic beverages. Through the previous four or five years I noticed that he never drank in his Florida bungalow, which was scantily furnished, and widely ventilated. In Florida, also, his disposition was always noticeably better than it was in his heavily furnished northern home.

"In the spring he had to stay for a time in my home, which had been thoroughly Dust-Sealed. So long as he was with us he had no desire to drink, and this observation taken together with the similar ones that I had made each year in Florida suggested to my allergy-conditioned mind that my father might be allergic to "house-dust," and that his craving for alcohol might be allergic.

"Without telling him why I was doing it I asked him to let me Dust-Seal his home; to which he agreed, being aware of the benefit of Dust-Sealing to the health of my family.

"I Dust-Sealed his home in March since which time he has drunk secretly only once—on the day when he had been working with an old untreated bedmattress. *The craving has disappeared, and it does not return when he drinks socially.*"

Dr. A., whose blood-pressure nearly ten years ago had reached a high point of 202/122, had reduced it to an average of 134.5/74, first through avoidance of pulse-accelerating foods and tobacco smoke, then through the control of "house dust" in his home with Dust-Seal and a plastic mattress cover.

Recently he undertook to test the dust-restraining efficiency of Dust-Sealed mattress ticking.

As a preliminary control he unzipped the plastic cover and drew it half-way down. Sleeping on the uncovered mattress three nights he found the blood pressure in the morning 158/80, 170/90 and 166/92 respectively. Thus, he proved again that there was something in his mattress which caused his high blood pressure. Then he had the mattress covered with the Dust-Sealed ticking, and his blood pressure after three successive nights was 120/76, 120/62 and 122/60.

The protective action of Dust-Seal is long lasting, not having yielded in rugs under constant use in a period of four and a half years after a thorough application. The treatment also extends the life of the fabrics.

Only one instance of allergic sensitivity to Dust-Seal itself has been reported; while several cases of such sensitivity to the dust-proof plastic covers have been observed.

House-dust sensitivity has been found to affect so large a proportion of the population, more than fifty percent, that manufacturers of bedding, rugs and upholstered furniture may be forced by popular demand to include Dust-Sealing as routine in the manufacture.

This idea was put in successful practice by the Ideal Toy Corporation in their manufacture of soft toys under the trade name "Algy." Asthmatic children known to be allergic to dust have had to be deprived of their Teddy Bears and dolls. Such children may use Dust-Sealed Algy toys without harm.

# (10)

## You Are Younger Than You Think

Most persons desire to prolong life as long as they can. Even when its pains are greater than its pleasures and comforts, most of us cling to life, and hope somehow that death will pass us by. Justice Oliver Wendell Holmes said, "To live is to function," and this is the sense in which most of us use the term life in our desire to prolong it.

How many of us think (only half seriously sometimes, to be sure) that we were better dead than blind or crippled or the victim of, say, leprosy? But few are the suicides among lepers.

You and I then wish for a postponement of the inescapable. We always do so with the hope that we'll be spared the common disabilities and restrictions of old age. So long as we are alive, we wish to "live."

And, "there's the rub." For the chance that you can escape those disabilities is pitifully slim. (Or I should say "has been slim," because now a much better chance has come within your choice as a result of what you have read in this book.)

Let us see which of the disabilities of "old age" are part of the normal biological aging process, and which are symptoms or effects of preventable disease.

Dr. Louis I. Dublin says that chronic nephritis, cerebral hemorrhage (stroke), diseases of the arteries and heart attacks are typical of the aging process.

This is indeed a discouraging conclusion. According to the authoritative statistics, these degenerative conditions are already observable in the age-group under 20. In fact, nearly three percent of the deaths occurring in that group are due to those conditions. Yet to say that those children die of "old age" would seem sufficiently to expose the *reductio ad absurdum.*

Experiences with the pulse-survey have thrown a bright, new light on this important question. They have shown us that the so-called "degenerative conditions" of old age are not inevitable.

Since the first reports ten years ago of the dietary control of high blood pressure by Dr. A Sumner Price and the author, the accumulated evidence has pointed more clearly to the change in the problem of that dread affliction.

The grin-and-bear-it counsel of passive resignation has now been replaced with the aggressive watch-words, "spot your allergens and eliminate them." Salvation for the hypersensitive now lies at his finger tips.

Two later reports greatly strengthen this conclusion. One came recently from Dr. Milo G. Meyer. It contained a list of 24 cured cases observed over a year. The second came from Dr. Walter Kempner, and it is of special interest because Dr. Kempner had applied the method of dietary restriction without realizing the anti-allergic effect of what he was doing.

He limited his patient's diet to rice, fruit-juices, sugar, vitamins and iron. Improvement (lowering of the pressure) was noted in about 60 percent of the cases. This selection of foods is known as the "rice-diet" and, in fact, Dr. Kempner attributed the improvement to the positive curative action of some mysterious constituent of rice.

However, it was not the eating of rice which lowered the blood-pressure, but the avoidance of all the commonest food-allergens. It has long been known that rice is one of the weakest and least common excitants of allergy. Among food-allergic persons 55 percent are not allergic to rice, fruit-juices and sugar, a figure close to the 60 percent reported by Dr. Kempner.

Statistics show that dietary control of heart attacks and high blood pressure with its customary involvement of the kidneys ("cardiovascular-renal disease") would extend the life span of a very great number of our people.

If 100,000 persons should be given the benefits of the pulse-survey from the age of say 16 years, and should adhere to their dietary restrictions, at least 25,000 of them would be living and well at 79, who otherwise would have died. Of all who now die between the ages of 50 and 60, about 40 percent could expect an extension of at least twenty years.

However, this program would not offer a mere extension of existence, but a continuation of active pleasurable *living*.

Here is a case in point.

Mrs. B. at 72 was a tired old woman spending much of

her time in bed, deprived of much of her social pleasure, and rather suspecting she would not be alive when her only son returned from Africa. That was ten years ago.

In her first interview with me she grasped the idea that in the new procedure she was not to play the passive role of the guinea-pig, but that of an active participant. She was to perform each test herself, and she was to be required to discuss each result and to know the reason for every decision.

She left looking tired but determined, and she pushed the tests to completion in three weeks. Her food-allergens were easily dispensable—milk, citrus fruit, carrot, beet, asparagus and onion.

Now, ten years later and what a change! The pains are forgotten; her unwanted fat is gone. That tired look in her eyes has been replaced with a sparkle of interest in life and living, in going and doing, and in the lesser questions of her wardrobe—a reliable sign that "old age" is still a good way off. Such is the picture of gracious aging in one who has escaped the claws of food-allergy. She was younger than she feared.

This method of allergen-avoidance which prevents death by heart attacks, stroke and uremic coma, also prevents the miseries and limitations of old age's other allergic conditions.

The migraine of middle life tends to lessen, or it may disappear, without diet control, but ordinarily old age carries with it the tired feeling, indigestion, constipation, nervousness and "stuffy" nose of earlier years.

To these are likely to be added neuralgic, rheumatic and arthritic pain and overweight, with the often associated aversion to physical activity. Still to be studied with the new method is gout, which is already under suspicion as a manifestation of allergy.

A common complaint that is akin to those just mentioned is that "aching back."

Old Dr. A. is delighted at the cessation of his recurring attacks of lumbago after he had completed his pulse-survey, but what really amazes him is his complete freedom from the formerly invariable stiffness when he takes a notion to defy his 70 years with a turn of mowing or snow-shoveling.

Not only has he no more of the stiffness, but the exercise brings the desired sense of physical well-being and an enhanced interest in the next mealtime.

High among the incidence of diseases of old age is cancer. One of the alleged disadvantages of a long life is the likelihood of one's arriving at the cancer-age. However, it is interesting and maybe significant that among men, the deaths from cancer per hundred between 90 and 100 are only one-third those between 60 and 70. And it is worth noting, I believe, that the same relationship exists in the case of diabetes, which is probably allergic.

These figures could suggest that most of those susceptible to these two conditions have died before they have reached 90.

The new knowledge of the importance, the cause and the methods of controlling and eliminating inheritable allergic disease gives us an encouraging view of the future happiness and longevity of mankind.

In the "promised land" of human freedom from inheritable disease, we can expect that both the normal aging process and the end of life itself will be painless.

The problem of old age will surely change when the new knowledge of food-allergy is put to universal use. Instead of planning for the care of the "aged," we shall have to find the work for them which they will certainly demand in their emancipation from the allergic handicap.

# (11)

## Explorations in Pulse-Dietary Therapy: Psychoneurosis, Alcoholism, Multiple Sclerosis

Your skin is the landscape of your body. It can exude inner health and beauty, or it can reflect the struggle of your system against its allergies.

The skin of some allergic persons is so sensitive to scratching that if you draw a line on it with a fingernail a pale welt bordered with a bright red flush appears. This phenomenon is called dermagraphism. The same thing happens with some other allergic persons' skin after a piece of ice is laid on it.

These allergic reactions are, of course, caused by secondary factors. The secondary factors may be physical or psychic. By physical I mean things like mechanical irritation (scratching, rubbing), heat, cold, sunlight and exertion.

It is an understandable error of symptomatic medicine that when such symptoms appear from such secondary factors, some allergists direct the patient merely to avoid the physical cause, as though it were primary.

It is a common experience that the normal or the

allergic person can be conditioned to tolerate these stimuli by repeated exposures to them if the repetitions do not follow at too short intervals. Thus by gradually lowering the temperature of the daily shower-bath you can arrive at a tolerance of the "cold" shower even at its winter temperature.

If allergic symptoms—usually hives or asthma—are excited by exposure to cold (water of air), the tolerance to cold can be increased in some of these persons, and, thereafter, exposure to cold within the limit of the increased tolerance will not cause these symptoms.

It is known that if you show "physical allergy" you are really allergic to some foods or inhalants.

If then the physical excitants of your allergic symptoms can act only upon your allergically abnormal tissues, you can expect that if you discover and avoid your allergic excitants, the so-called "physical allergy" will no longer exist.

The truth of this is shown in a case of bronchial asthma in a young woman who, before the dietary diagnosis, suffered severe asthmatic attacks on exposure to cold air, and also under *excitement*. Only four foods caused acceleration of her pulse, and when these were avoided her asthma ceased and excitement and exposure to cold air no longer brought on attacks.

This illustration of the psychic influence (excitement) in "food-allergy" brings us to the consideration of the "psychic" secondary factor. This is more important to our understanding of many medical phenomena than the several "physical" factors.

Warren T. Vaughan in his book *Practice of Allergy* cites

a number of cases out of his own observations, and some contributed by "friends" that show the "psychogenic" factors that start allergic symptoms. For example:

1. A young woman who suffered hives only at widely separated occasions, at each of which she was emotionally upset by the distasteful attentions of a suitor.

2. A man who had three outbreaks of hives, each one after emotional disturbance caused by his wife's unfaithfulness.

Vaughan did not apply the (at that time unknown) pulse-dietary method of detecting the food-allergic primary excitants of the hives in these two cases. Hence, the emotional disturbances seemed to be the only cause of the attacks.

A third case contributed by Dr. French K. Hansel reveals clearly the true relations:

Hansel's patient was allergic to wheat. This caused migraine when eaten liberally, but did not if eaten "in moderation." However, even when wheat was being eaten in a "customary amount" an attack of migraine could be brought on by an "emotional upset." Total avoidance of wheat was followed by cessation of all migraine attacks.

A not unrelated example of allergic reaction was cited by *Business Week* in February 1982. It seems that halothane, an anesthetic gas, had caused catastrophic (that means fatal) destruction of the liver in some surgical patients. It turned out that those who suffered acute hepatitis in varying degrees after surgery during which the gas was administered to them never responded the first time. It was always a second or third use of the gas that did the damage.

This is much like the several cases I've cited of people who can tolerate a food allergen once a week without a problem. But a more frequent contact with the food allergen produced a return of the old symptoms.

The highly important lesson to be drawn from this discussion of the secondary factors in food-allergy is that these factors are effective only on the basis of an already existing food-allergy irritation of the tissues.

The noted Spanish allergist B. Sanchez-Cuenca has named this irritable state of the tissues "allergic tension."

In short, these experiences suggest that allergic symptoms are never purely psychogenic. The instances that seem to contradict this conclusion have probably not been adequately studied with the specific methods that are now available.

Psychologic influences not only may precipitate allergic symptoms; they may paradoxically, also do away with them altogether—if only for a limited time. This is illustrated in the following case I observed:

A man had suffered severe migraine attacks at about biweekly intervals for many years. These came with spells of dizziness, tiredness, indigestion, and more recently a recurring blind spot in one eye caused by an internal "hive" on the retina.

He was advised on several occasions to take a West Indian cruise "for his health." Each time, all of these allergic symptoms disappeared a few days after he set out. But they came back again in full force not long after his return. This man was later found to be allergic to all but one food; hence his varied diet on board ship could not have been limited, by chance, to nonallergic foods.

The only circumstances to which the sudden complete freedom from his allergic symptoms could be credited were the change in his environment and associates, and his release from numerous pressing responsibilities, these being replaced by daily changing programs of recreation—in short, primarily psychologic influences.

The fundamentally allergic nature of the man's symptoms was finally demonstrated through the pulse-dietary method. His condition was relieved by sympathectomy followed by observance of a moderately restricted diet.

The cases I've cited are representative of many similar ones. They occur constantly in the experience of medical practitioners and specialists, especially neurologists and psychiatrists.

There are two general classifications into which the psychiatrist can place the great majority of his patients. Into the first goes the psychoneurotic patient described as being in contact with reality, and into the second goes the psychotic individual who is described as living in and dealing with unreality. The latter has created and moved into a world of phantasy with its delusions and hallucinations, which he has great difficulty in distinguishing from real life. Such are the insane.

An interesting case in the first classification is a typical one of neurasthenia in a woman for whom the psychoanalytic treatment failed, but who has been freed of her trouble by anti-allergic treatment.

K. T., a woman of 26 years, came for consultation in what she said was her final effort to obtain medical help. If this failed, she was contemplating suicide. A valued employee of a large insurance company in New York, she had been sent to psychiatrists, and finally to a sanatorium for mental ailments, where she remained for two months under psychoanalytic treatment. Her symptoms were recurrent nausea, constipation, neuralgia, "fluttery heart," marked abnormal tiredness, severe attacks of dizziness, weeping spells and psychic depression. The psychiatric diagnosis was "nervous and emotional instability—incurable."

The diversions at the sanatorium caused a moderate improvement in her general health. She put on weight and felt less depressed. However, the attacks of dizziness continued, and on her return they interfered so seriously with her work that she faced the loss of her position.

Her physician had recommended injections of a bacterial vaccine, and she noticed that her symptoms, especially the dizziness, were always worse after an injection. It was this observation that caused her to consult me. When I explained the possibly allergic cause of her illness she eagerly agreed to try the pulse-dietary procedure.

As soon as she had begun to avoid her chief food-allergens, all of her symptoms ceased. However, several important foods later showed themselves as minor allergens that had to be avoided, leaving her ultimately with an inadequate diet. She had to resort to a sympathectomy, after which the list of her food-allergens was so greatly reduced that an entirely satisfactory diet became available.

Here is the considerable list of the food-allergens that were identified previous to the nerve operation. The items in capital letters are those which could be eaten in unlimited quantity after the operation without the slightest perceptible allergic reaction. As soon as she was sure that she was cured she married, and is now the happy mother of two daughters.

| Group 1 (major) | Group 2 (medium) | Group 3 (minor) |
|---|---|---|
| BEEF | tomato | CANE-SUGAR |
| orange | RICE | potato |
| WHEAT | OAT | banana |
| grapefruit | RYE | STRAWBERRY |
| lemon | CORN | |
| PLUM | coffee | |
| | ONION | |

After she had made the pulse-survey following her operation she became aware of a previously unidentified allergen which caused moderate spells of dizziness. This she herself discovered to be something in the local water supply.

There have been other reports of such cases.

Recently that particular allergen figured in an episode which should impress any reader who may still suspect a psychologic factor in this woman's symptoms. One evening she sent John to the refrigerator for a glass of her distilled water which has never affected her. About ten minutes thereafter she had a short dizzy spell.

"John are you sure that was the distilled water you brought me?"

"Sure thing—why?"

"Will you please check, John? I'm curious." John found the distilled water bottle on the table—empty. The bottle in the refrigerator which he had used contained tap water.

The patient reports one interesting difference between her present accidentally or sometimes deliberately induced attacks and those experienced formerly. "Now," she says, "I suffer no depression because I know the cause of the attack."

The pulse-dietary tests should be made the first step in

the examination of every patient being studied for mental defects.

The use of the procedure of psychoanalysis would seem to represent a modern refinement of our old acquaintance—symptomatic treatment. Moreover, it is reasonable to assume that nearly all of those patients who are now being treated with that method are in need of the new antiallergic treatment with which their chances of permanent recovery seem excellent.

My purpose is not to condemn the practice of psychoanalysis, but to call attention to what may be the primary physical causes of the mental effects which the psychiatrist treats on the mental plane. If the primary cause is physical its treatment should be physical, and in such a case psychiatric treatment can be harmful as a primary measure.

If for any of the reasons that have been mentioned the antiallergic procedure should fail to discover all of the physical excitants of the mental or nervous symptoms, or if the avoidance of those excitants should seem impracticable, then one may resort to the psychiatric technics, though, one should think, with dampened enthusiasm.

Many a victim of allergic psychoneurosis wakes on the morning after heavy indulgence in one or more of his food allergens with a sensation of anxiety or even fright, or in a state of angry irritability accompanied with fatigue.

In either case he usually does not recall what he ate the night before, but tries, often with success, to remember anything he could be anxious or frightened about, or anybody who had offended him. But our associates and their acts do not *make* us angry. It is our food-allergy that upsets our equanimity and arouses our anger, and we take it out on our associates.

After the allergy is eliminated we find ourselves simply incapable of anger, even under heavy provocation.

Experience with the pulse-dietary means of disease-prevention has brought out the important conclusion that irritability is not a normal human quality, but a preventable manifestation of idioblaptic allergy.

The first two instances of pronounced irritability that came to my particular notice should interest those who are concerned with the problems of industrial and domestic human relations.

Mr. K., the epileptic man who has been mentioned earlier as having induced a seizure by smoking, is the chief of a group of employees in a large manufacturing company. Long after he was sure that his epilepsy was a thing of the past, at his discretion, he reported with astonishment that whereas he had had constant difficulties with his men on account of his marked irritability, his relations with them since he began to control his allergy had become entirely satisfactory. He had "lost the *tendency* to become irritable," and he asked whether this tendency might be an allergic symptom.

Mrs. B., aged 50, head of a group of employees in a large pharmaceutical company, could not "get along with her subordinates on account of her snappish disposition." She wondered that her husband did not leave her, and sincerely mourned her "uncontrolled temper."

Her chief allergic symptoms were constant headache, marked physical tiredness and neuralgia, all of which vanished as soon as she began to avoid her two pulse-accelerating foods, wheat and pork. Several months later she told me that her irritability had departed with the symptoms, and she asked whether that was also "allergic." Through the succeeding five years of my communication with her she positively maintained that she had entirely, "lost the capacity to become irritated," either at work or at home.

It seems reasonable to assume that the cause of irritability and of "tantrums" in the child or adult is one and the same. At any rate Dr. Susan Dees in Duke University has reported evidence of the allergic nature of tantrums in children.

A six year old girl was the victim of violent tantrums. She was found by her physician to be pulse-sensitive to so many foods that the nerve operation was required. After that only one substance (something in "hot-dog") brought on a spell of tantrum in the child. Otherwise she is a quite normally behaved girl.

## Alcoholism

The most easily understood definition of "alcoholism" in the sense in which it is to be discussed here is that it represents a *craving* for alcoholic beverage as distinguished from a pleasurable taste for it.

The alcoholic person is a *compulsive* drinker. This condition is recognized by authorities as a symptomatic entity, the diagnostic signs of which were recently listed in a radio discussion as follows:

1. Drinking alone.
2. Drinking in the morning.
3. "Black-out" episodes.

Not all compulsive drinkers indulge to the point of actual drunkenness. The radio speaker, an outstanding authority on this matter, stated that "alcoholism cannot be cured." He explained that although many subjects are able to abstain entirely from alcoholic drinks, none can drink socially without yielding to the craving which persists. However, at the time he was speaking a report was being prepared for publication in which the specific, allergic cause of alcoholism was being demonstrated, and with it the means of its "cure." (See case report of Mr. X., p. 130.)

## Multiple Sclerosis

Multiple sclerosis is a progressive paralytic disease of the central nervous system. It is rated as "incurable." In fact, one professor of neurology, after he had read the report of many years of freedom from the disease produced by three widely separated physicians with the use of the pulse-dietary and other antiallergic procedures, objected in all seriousness to the favorable report of the preventative treatment, on the ground that no else had succeeded with other kinds of treatment in restoring victims of multiple sclerosis "to a physical and economic state which is functionally useful."

This criticism suggests that if the reported cases were "cured" they were not subjects of multiple sclerosis.

One is led by such an attitude to wonder what the researchers in multiple sclerosis are looking for if they will not believe that a prevention of it is possible.

After Dr. Milo G. Meyer of Michigan City, Indiana, had led the way with his successful use of antiallergic prevention in multiple sclerosis, I was most pleased to have the opportunity to follow him with a case of multiple sclerosis who had been given up as hopeless by the authorities at the Neurological Institute in New York City.

At least those experts had no doubt that the man had multiple sclerosis; and the patient himself, now at his job for several years in a machine shop, and occasionally driving a truck, is convinced that he has been restored to a functionally and economically useful state.

The immediate cause of the man's disease was his allergy to cigarettes, which he smoked end to end through the day. He was not allergic to the common foods, though his pulse was affected by some ingredient of a locally produced sausage.

A smoking test of only two inhaled puffs carried his pulse to 92 in five minutes, whereupon he swore off the weed for his life (in the two senses). Five days later he could get down stairs without holding the bannister, and he could play ball with his son's bat, which previously he could not even hold up. There has been no recurrence of the disease in the subsequent four years.

It is one of the many mysterious facts concerning the newly defined allergic disease that in the victims of multiple sclerosis the allergy itself is regularly present *in its lease severe degree*. Only one of the twenty cases that have been examined with the pulse-dietary method has been sensitive to so many foods as to need a sympathectomy, whereas 20 percent of the usual cases with other symptoms (migraine, asthma, eczema, etc.) require that operation. And about 80 percent of severely affected epileptics have needed it.

These facts have been brought to the attention of the society which professes a special interest in multiple sclerosis; but thus far the directors have not seen fit to put the life-saving procedure to work for the benefit of the otherwise hopelessly affected thousands.

In fact, the medical advisory board of the society in regular meetings were unanimously of the opinion that the preventative pulse-dietary procedure is without merit. They did not consider it necessary to *try* the method before condemning it.

# (12)

## "You Don't Catch Colds—
## You Eat Them"

> "We know more about radioactivity than
> we do about colds."
> —Official U.S. Government booklet,
> *Survival Under Atomic Attack*

What do you know about *your* colds?

Outstanding among the items of "knowlege" concerning common cold are the wide misconceptions about the most prevalent of all infections. These misconceptions are held and spread not only by the laity, but also by some members of the medical profession.

Among the misconceptions is one which says common cold may be caused by exposure to drafts or changes in room-temperature, or by fatigue, or the excessive use of alcoholic beverages, or the breathing of irritating dust, or by various bacteria normally inhabiting the respiratory tract.

The error in all of these assumptions was neatly exposed in the report by Drs. Paul and Freese of their investigation of common cold in the small community of Longyear City in Spitsbergen.

In Longyear City common colds are not prevalent in the fall, winter and spring as they are in continental communities, but they occur in epidemic form each summer. These annual epidemics begin about 48 hours following the arrival in late May of the first boat from the Norwegian mainland, from which the city has been isolated throughout the fall, winter and spring. About 90 percent of the 507 inhabitants, that is, all the susceptible persons, are ultimately affected.

From this account of the occurrence of common cold in Longyear City the following conclusions reasonably appear:

1. Common cold in Longyear City cannot be caused by exposure to drafts, changes of temperature, fatigue, indulgence in alcohol.

2. Common cold in Longyear City cannot be caused by bacteria normally inhabiting the respiratory tract of the people there. This second conclusion is supported by the finding of the investigators that the bacteria present in the mouths of the inhabitants in the cold months of isolation are not significantly different from those present in the summer when colds are prevalent.

Contrast this negative result with the fact that in bacterial infections such as diphtheria, pneumonia, scarlet fever, typhoid fever and the others the respective causative bacteria are regularly demonstrable in the infected tissues, and usually as the predominant microorganism.

3. Common cold must be infectious, each affected person having acquired the infection from another affected person. The particular infectious micro-organism of common cold is brought to the city in late May by the first boatload of passengers, and it dies out there in the late summer.

When competent investigators consistently fail to cultivate special bacteria from the infected tissues in an evidently infectious disease, this usually points to some virus or, much less commonly, Rickettsia,* as the infectious agent.

The well-known experiments of Dochez and his associates, and those of P. H. Long and his co-workers pointed directly to a virus as the cause of the common cold.

Among the qualified medical scientists, then, there is a general impression that the exciting cause of common cold is of the nature of the ultramicroscopic virus. For this reason it is of interest to acquaint ourselves with the peculiarities of these minute enemies of man.

The viruses are not nearly so susceptible as the bacteria to the common antiseptics, or to some of the new wonder-drugs. The sulfa-drugs and penicillin have been found useless in the viral infections studied so far.

The viruses invade the tissues more deeply than do the bacteria, entering even the nucleus of the body-cells. Within the tissue-cells the viruses are safe from the destructive or at least neutralizing action of a protective serum because serum is unable to penetrate the cells quickly enough, if at all, to exert a curative effect.

It is for these reasons that the serum-treatment of rabies and polio (both viral infections) has failed, and that the prospect of any such treatment of common cold would be discouraging even if the cold-virus had been cultivated, or if an easily available cold-susceptible animal were known in which a protective serum could be produced.

From these considerations it is seen that you cannot

*Rickettsia: microorganisms discovered by Dr. Ricketts, of a size between virus and bacteria. Typhus fever is caused by Rickettsia.

hope for a solution to the physically and economically serious problem of common cold in drugs or injections.

Antiseptic gargles and sprays and medicated tablets are only palliative at best, and the first two are believed sometimes to help spread the infection. The benefits of vaccines, vitamins, laxatives and exercise are slight.

*However, the problem has at last been solved, and in a most unexpected way.* The first step was taken by an experienced investigator of medical biology, Arthur P. Locke.

Dr. Locke observed differences among rabbits in their susceptibility to the germs of pneumonia (pneumococus). He discovered that the more resistant rabbits were those that recovered their normal temperatures after a brief immersion in cool water within an optimal range of time—not too quickly nor too slowly.

He saw in this observation a possible explanation of the well-known fact that some persons never have colds while most of us have one or more every year; and his studies in human beings brilliantly confirmed his anticipations.

Dr. Locke could show that persons who are not susceptible to common cold recover more quickly from violent exercise, and from the effect of breathing air containing five percent carbonic acid gas than persons who are cold-susceptible.

Locke proved, in other words, that the cold-susceptible person suffers from a general handicap that renders him susceptible to an infection to which the physically fit person is immune. Physical fitness in the sense of Locke is not, of course, synonymous with superior muscular development, since many athletic people are very susceptible to colds.

The nature of the physical handicap postulated by Locke was revealed in my statistical study of common cold and of food-allergy in 825 employees at Lederle Laboratories.

I began my study on the basis of a mistaken conclusion. For several years I had gargled faithfully with a powerfully antiseptic Australian oil, and in that period I had had definitely fewer and milder colds than ever before.

Throughout my adult life I had gone to bed for five or six days three or four times each year while the cold germs travelled in their devilishly leisurely tempo from my throat to the uttermost reaches of sinuses and bronchial tubes, wringing water out of me at every step; while lately my annual quota was one attack, with only one or two really bad days. I credited the improvement to the oil.

At last having some spare time I staged a large-scale gargling experiment among 400 cold-susceptibles through four months of fall and winter. To my disgust, the control group who did *not* gargle had fewer colds than those who did!

The intuitive (?) solution to the mystery came from Mrs. Coca, my severest critic. She offered, "Maybe you have fewer colds because you have been controlling your food-allergy!" And the material was ready for the test of her suggestion. We began the next day.

Of the 825 employees, 99 (Locke's 12 percent) had not had a cold in three years. Fifty-two of these were interviewed, and about eighty percent (and most of their parents) were found to be nonallergic, whereas about ninety percent of the cold-susceptible group of fifty-one persons were allergic.

It was evident upon that statistical finding that if one

is free from allergy one is likely also to be free from common cold.

This striking relationship of "food-allergy" to susceptibility to colds was then confirmed by Dr. Locke and his associates in an extensive study of the students at Stevens College for women at Columbia, Missouri. The physical handicap of Locke turns out to be the effects of "food-allergy." Thus one is justified in entertaining the possibility that since in the large majority of instances, "food-allergy" is the most important predisposing cause of common cold, the personal or genetic elimination of "food-allergy" will be followed by freedom from colds.

This possibility has already been realized in a number of "food-allergic" persons who were formerly very susceptible to colds, not only as to frequency—several each year—but also as to severity—one to several weeks confinement to bed or house. After avoidance of all allergic food-poisons was practised, they've had no more colds. This, in spite of continued close association with persons severely affected with colds.

The predisposition to colds is not an ineradicable handicap in the "food-allergic" person. It comes and goes with our allergic episodes, and we have only to show the door to our allergies through the use of the pulse-key in order to bid farewell to the commonest and most expensive of all infections.

We are now able to summarize the problem of common cold as follows:

1. Your common cold is not caused by exposure to drafts, chilling or changes of temperature. However, once

the infection is established and is full-blown, such exposures do aggravate the condition, sometimes markedly.

2. Your common cold is an infectious disease probably caused by a virus of low virulence (Locke), which is incapable of causing death by itself, although it often prepares the way for other much more serious, even fatal infections such as pneumonia.

3. Your common cold can develop only after association with a person who carried the infective virus. However, the term "association" applies also in those frequent occasions when the susceptible individual breathes air in a place that has recently been visited by an infected person. Under favorable conditions the air may contain living and infectious cold-virus. Those favorable conditions in the case of other agents of respiratory infection are cold and humidity, both of which are commonly prevalent in fall, winter and spring.

(It was observed many years ago by Richard P. Strong and Oscar Teague that bacteria sprayed into a dry, warm atmosphere died in a few minutes, whereas if they were sprayed into a cold, humid atmosphere they remained alive, suspended in the air for as long as an hour and a half.)

4. The virus of common cold has not been cultivated; hence there is no immunizing vaccine for your common cold. The acquired immunity to the virus that is present at the time of recovery from an attack is relatively very brief (weeks' or months' duration).

5. The virus of your common cold is not perceptibly affected by antiseptics in the usual concentrations, as in gargles or sprays, nor by the newer drugs, so far as is known.

6. If you are free from "food-allergy" you will enjoy an absolute natural immunity to the virus of common cold.

# (13)

# Beauty at Your Fingertips

A number of allergic conditions offend the sensibilities of society, and cause humiliation in those who suffer from them. Some have been discussed elsewhere in this book. Overweight, underweight and stammering (which is sometimes unpleasantly aggravated by the accompanying facial twitching) can be corrected through the procedure of allergen avoidance.

These disabilities are annoying, but there are others still more distressing to many sensitive men as well as women. These are the disfiguring allergic affections of the skin.

Mr. F., a prominent business man tolerated his occasional headaches, his neuralgia, tiredness and indigestion with resignation. What drove him to the specialists' offices was his red, scaly fingers, which caused him acute embarrassment when meeting strangers.

"I hate having to shake hands with new business acquaintances," he complained. "I know some of them suspect the eruption as catching."

Two weeks after his first interview with me he reported that the skin was generally clear, and two years later the hands were still quite clear though slightly pinker than normal. He had been avoiding yeast (as in bread and beer), and also all meats excepting fowl. When he made his last test of beef it was immediately followed by a "bad outbreak of the eczema." That lesson seems to have convinced him.

Before Mr. F. came for the pulse-survey he had consulted a well-known New York allergist who skin-tested him and curiously reported him *not* allergic to beef, lamb, nor yeast. On the other hand the skin-test would have him allergic to chocolate, which he eats without the slightest disturbance of skin or pulse. Again, we see that whereas the skin-test is indispensable in hay fever, it is unreliable in food-allergy.

The skin which is properly rated by medical science as an important organ, and not merely a protective covering, is variously affected by food-allergy. A common effect of the disease is some interference with the capillary circulation which, for one thing, deprives the skin of its natural ruddy color, leaving a sallow, "pasty" hue, even in warm weather with some persons; and this depletion of the blood supply may adversely affect the hair and nails as well as the sweat and oil glands.

Mr. A. who has been a life-long victim of numerous severe allergic symptoms was afflicted every winter with chapped hands and face (especially the lips) and cracked finger nails. The fissured, thickened skin at the sides of his finger nails bled unless they were protected with collodion. His feet were constantly cold and were occasionally frostbitten. His skin was always sallow. It was also excessively oily, presenting a constant succession of blackheads, some of enormous bulk.

This cheerless picture is rounded out by the fact that, at 66, Mr. A.'s hair was rapidly deserting him.

One year later he had controlled his food-allergy, and the picture was immediately reversed. His skin became pink, his hands and lips do not chap nor crack in winter, his nails remain smooth and also pink, his feet stay warm in the coldest weather; there is no excessive oil in the skin, and blackheads are rare.

Not only is he losing no more hair, but actually there is very slow growth of *new* hair—which is black. It seems reasonable to suppose that the correction of the allergy may have halted the circulatory starvation of the hair-follicles and the loss of hair. However, one need not be so optimistic as to expect the new method to cure baldness, which by the way, is known to be due in some cases to causes other than allergy. Once the hair-follicle (root) is starved to death there can be no recovery.

Mr. V., at the end of a rather strenuous but faithfully conducted pulse-survey, which revealed sixteen food-allergens, found himself free-from his headaches, asthma and tiredness.

One month later he reported with evident satisfaction that his acne also was gone, and with it the very annoying excessive oiliness of his skin.

Miss M.'s case has been described in the discussion of overweight. One of the gratifying results of her pulse-survey was the complete healing of her "constantly cracked nails."

Mrs. Mc., a dancer, could correct her pallid complexion with cosmetic art, but she was concerned over the rough patch on her left cheek. It did not rate as an eczema; it was merely an unsightly blemish to her—something she got from mother and dad.

Mrs. Mc. did not ask for the pulse-survey on account of her complexion, but because of recurrent attacks of "blindness." Those attacks ceased after the completion of the tests, and so have her fears; but I imagine that secretly she takes greater satisfaction from the improved color of her skin, and the now faultless surface of her left cheek.

The runny nose can spoil one's appearance whatever its excitant-cause; but the first instance in illustration has the added interest of being caused by a cosmetic material—lipstick.

Vivacious little Miss P. had a ready smile and a friendly word for all of us in the office. She was expecting to marry her navy officer a year hence, and her cup should have been running over with anticipated happiness. But I had not noticed her nose, which was forever running over, nor her secret unhappiness, which was caused by her continual tiredness and recurring headaches.

So I was astonished when she came to me one morning looking forlorn and discouraged.

"Will you help me?" she begged. "I am worried about myself—I'm afraid I'm no good; I'll just be a drag on my husband. And look at my nose!"

"Cold?" I asked.

"No, it's this way most of the time, and I think it's worse whenever I am in company."

The pulse-survey was quickly and luckily completed;

the single culprit was egg, and avoidance of it was immediately followed by the disappearance of tiredness and headaches.

One day she came in sniffling and dejected. "When did this begin?" I questioned.

"A little while ago."

"How is the pulse?"

"92."

"No egg?"

"No egg."

"What have you been doing?" After some thought she replied with a question. "Could this possibly be due to lipstick? I put it on just an hour ago."

"I don't know." I said. "Let's see; take it off." Within an hour after she had done a careful job of cleaning, her pulse was down to her normal rate, and her nose was dry.

The lipstick she had used was not her regular brand (Woolworth), but an expensive, widely known brand name. I succeeded in obtaining the twelve different ingredients of the product from the company, and easily identified number 6 as the trouble-maker. Application of that substance caused a rapid pulse and the runny nose. The Woolworth product did not affect her at all.

I reported the results to the manufacturers, suggesting that they try to get along without the offending ingredient. They refused, saying that they had had "no other complaints."

J. F. models in clay. Imagine a clay-modeler trying to contend with a runny nose! Before her emancipation through the pulse-survey she spoke as though through an inexpertly applied gag. Add to these disturbances her headaches, tiredness and constipation, and you have the picture of a case of so-called "psychosomatic disorders."

The pulse-survey incriminated lamb, chicken, egg, potato, tomato, citrus fruit, chocolate, coffee and tea. Egg was the most vicious offender. A single indulgence was followed by an "attack" that resembled a bad cold and lasted five or six days.

This is the tenth year since she learned how, with her fingertips and her watch, to regulate her health and keep her nose dry.

# (14)

## Some Problems
## You May Encounter

I have been advised to include this chapter by my former laboratory associate (E. L. C.), who has had much experience in the interpretation of pulse-dietary records, and who has read the first portion of the manuscript. She says, "The pulse-survey as it is described is made to sound easier than it is; some readers will try to apply it to themselves, and they will be disillusioned when they encounter some of its difficulties."

This criticism is fair, and it has support in the fact that some lay-people already have read my technical monograph and have indeed applied the method to themselves or their relatives. They succeeded too, but only because the monograph discusses the difficulties fully, and, more important, because they are endowed with conspicuously more than average openmindedness and determination.

Some of the difficulties that one could encounter are due to misunderstandings. Thus, some persons cannot see any reason for counting the pulse *before* eating; some have snacks or soft drinks, or chew gum between meals without making any kind of record; some report having eaten soup or goulash or salad without noting the ingredients.

One man, after assuring me that he understood the principle of the *five single food meals*, applied it in the following manner: He ate five substantial meals to each of which he added the particular food to be tested. To my complaint that he had misunderstood the instructions he huffed, "I don't think you know what you're doing," and signed off.

But there are several intrinsic difficulties attaching to the pulse-survey which will now be described.

### The Carry-over

This phenomenon is seen in both the pulse and the symptoms. When C. G. ate wheat, which was the only cause of her hives, her elevated pulse-rise and the hives persisted for two and a half days after she had stopped the wheat. In some persons the reaction may last five or six days. This carry-over effect often interferes with the interpretation of any other tests made in that period.

A disturbing feature of the carry-over effect is its erratic course. There is not a gradual descent from the initial high point. Indeed, the initial rise is sometimes substantially exceeded on the next day. J. G.'s first test of wheat (the major cause of his migraine) pushed his pulse to 90 twice in that day. In the evening the count dropped to a normal 74, but the next morning (although he ate no wheat) it shot suddenly to 100, quickly falling again to 74.

## Temporarily Lost Sensitivity (Delayed Reaction)

This remarkable phenomenon, which is mentioned elsewhere in this book, is often confusing. It has been described by other writers, but I did not know of it until it appeared in an asthmatic young woman in her first test or orange. She had not eaten the fruit in recent weeks, so she celebrated her renewed acquaintance with it by continuing the test at each meal for two days.

On the second day headache began, and her pulse rose rapidly to 104. She was then "full of orange," and her reaction lasted three days. Fortunately she had not made any new tests in those two days and so was able to recognize the orange as the cause of her prolonged reaction.

This experience illustrates the necessity of testing each new food at least twice within two, or better three days. The longer the interval since the previous eating of a food the more often it should be retested, because the temporarily lost sensitivity is longer getting back.

Let us pause here to consider the question of the possible appearance of *new* food-sensitivities in adults.

We do not become allergic to a particular food that has always agreed with us by eating unusually large quantities of it, or eating it more often. The foods to which we are allergic were predetermined in our inheritance, and the allergy is established soon after our first exposure to them. Indeed, some observations suggest that effective exposure to food proteins may be had before birth by way of the mother's blood.

However, it seems illogical to warn expectant mothers not to eat "too much" (whatever that may mean) of any one food for fear of making her baby allergic to it. If the child is destined by inheritance to become allergic to a certain food it would appear to matter little whether the first exposure to that food occurs before birth or shortly thereafter.

## The Major and Minor Allergens

Some allergens are more powerful than others. What is meant by "more powerful" and less powerful—major and minor—allergens?

K. T., one of our most instructive cases was found in the first survey to be allergic to wheat, beef, citrus fruit and plum family.

After avoiding these foods she was quite well for a few months, but then suffered a gradual return of her dizziness, tiredness and other symptoms which were again dispelled by avoidance of the other cereals, tomato, coffee and onion. The next interval of freedom lasted about one month, when another crop of allergens emerged—cane sugar, potato, banana, berries and aluminum.

The word "emerged" is used to indicate not new sensitivities, but the appearance of already existing weak sensitivities which had been covered up by more powerful ones. It may be said that the effect of the major allergens on the susceptible tissues renders these tolerant for a time toward the much weaker action of the minor ones.

Wheat is usually major over rice, rye and oat, but corn is independent of the other cereals; that is, many persons must avoid all cereals but corn, while some can at all cereals except corn. Sensitivity to cane sugar is frequent, and seems to run rather with corn-sensitivity.

It is the minor allergen that can be eaten at intervals of a week or more with impunity (Dr. Summer Price).

Some persons seem to be affected only by minor allergens; at least some are sensitive to only one or two allergens, which can be eaten safely at intervals. The same food may be "major" in one person, but "minor" in another.

The several instances of sensitivity to aluminum that I have seen became apparent only after the major excitants had been identified and avoided. But the first report of such sensitivity came from Drs. Tchijevsky and Tchijevskaya in Moscow, concerning a long-standing case of colitis in which aluminum appeared to be the sole allergen, for the colitis was "cured" by a mere change from aluminum cooking utensils to enamel or glassware.

### Sensitivity to a Large Number of Important Foods

I will discuss this difficulty in connection with the conservative sympathectomy. This has been found to be a simple and dependable way out of that otherwise intolerable dilemma. It is the recognition of the nature of the difficulty that will stump the amateur when he first meets it; in which case he may gracefully acknowledge his need of expert assistance.

### Inhalants

This difficulty I have already discussed elsewhere. I have a not very scientific impression that the inhalants, excepting tobacco, are likely to be minor allergens, which begin to bite after the pulse is nearly (but not quite) stabilized. In this situation one should suspect bedding-dust, and should note whether the pulse tends to be higher just before rising than it was before retiring.

### The Public and the Principles

May I add that I am in favor of encouraging the public to study the principles and difficulties of the pulse-survey, and to *try* to apply them in the solving of their own allergic ailments. Sooner or later these principles must be taught in the high schools so that each graduate may become the custodian of his own health.

To the beginner, layman or doctor, who makes up his mind to master the new technic, I recommend careful study of my monograph, especially the chapter on Practical Management and the six succeeding chapters.

Finally I would again draw special attention to the most dependable evidence that the survey has been successful.

You will know that you have achieved success if, under the daily fourteen-count routine, the highest count is within one, or at the most two, pulse beats of the same figure every day for five days—and if you are without symptoms.

# (15)

# Breaking Through
# the Nerve Barrier

Often I am asked, "Is it possible for the pulse survey to fail?" The answer is that there are exceptions to the rules, but that a way to cope with these exceptions has been found.

You have a sympathetic nervous system. It consists of a double chair of massive nerve tissue, with nerve connections extending up and down the right and left sides of the spinal column from the neck to the end of the spine. It performs its duties independently of your brain and spinal cord; hence its other name, the "autonomic" nervous system.

The tasks which your sympathetic nerves perform appear to be local. For example, the paralysis or removal of one or more of the sympathetic nerve-ganglia stops perspiration, not of the whole skin, but only of the area of skin supplied by the particular nerves involved in the operation.

Removal of a sympathetic nerve-ganglion or injections of alcohol into it has been sometimes followed by the lasting improvement of a number of different disabilities of unknown cause. Among these is hypertension.

The long-range results of sympathectomy alone in hypertension are pitifully disappointing—only about six percent of the patients maintaining improvement after 3 to 5 years, according to a recent report. Nevertheless the operation in a dreadfully radical form that costs 6 to 10 weeks of hospitalization, and 6 to 10 weeks of "convalescence" is in reputable standing among the medical fraternity. It is justified as being "better than nothing."

Because they accept the theory of the local functions of the sympathetic nerves, most surgeons believe that the favorable effects of sympathectomy in the few cases of hypertension result from some local influence upon the kidneys. The kidneys are suspected as the origin of that disease.

This concept of local action of the sympathetic nerves is contradicted by the experience of every surgeon who has used the lumbar operation (removal of sympathetic ganglia in the back at about the level of the kidneys). These surgeons all report that if the patient has been a sufferer from recurrent headaches, the headaches promptly disappear after the operation. This is true even when the hypertension is unchanged or actually increases.

Here, then, is an established fact that cannot be made to fit into the theory of a local action of the operation; it points instead to a constitutional effect which is consistent with other indications that *recurrent headaches of all degrees are practically always allergic.*

The surgeons were and indeed are still unaware of this fact. Strangely, they will refuse to use the operation for the relief of recurrent headache, however severe, unless it is associated with hypertension.

I began my study of the antiallergic effect of sympathectomy after I had a hunch. My hunch was mothered by my own persistent case of allergy.

The symptoms I suffered included, besides all the eleven common ones, the frightening one of frequent, temporary loss of memory. Hypertension had not yet arrived—it was due a few months later.

I had learned to escape all of those symptoms by mere avoidance of the "food-allergens," but had not learned to live contentedly on beef alone—*the only food to which I was not allergic.*

My hunch was unsteadily balanced on two legs: 1) I knew that my trouble was allergic, and 2) I was convinced that hypertension is a consequence of allergy.

I had just learned that sympathectomy is without any effect in experimental hypertension induced in animals with mechanical means. So I reasoned that if human hypertension is sometimes relieved by sympathectomy (fortunately I did not know how seldom), and if experimental hypertension is not, then the favorable effect of the operation could be against the primary case of high blood pressure in man—that is, against the allergy.

The hunch had barely been born when I reached for the telephone and located a former student who had become a master of the art of surgery and was experienced in sympathectomies.

He listened to me. Then he announced that since my idea was new and unblessed by medical authority, I would have to accept full responsibility in writing. My enthusiasm at my possible relief from the operation was not diminished by his doubt, so I went to the operating table full of impatience to get to the first test meal after it, and quite forgot the possible risk I knew was connected with the procedure.

The result was a marvelous confirmation of my expectations. Within 48 hours I was eating without any restrictions, and was free from all allergic symptoms. Secondary problems of serious importance were to develop later. I will get to these presently.

Five more of my patients at the time were allergically in the same situation. All foods, or nearly all, affected them. When they learned the operation had immediate beneficial effects with me they all asked for it. The surgeon was willing to oblige—again on my responsibility. Trouble followed almost immediately.

The three epileptics among them suffered as many seizures as before. The psychoneurotic girl was as dizzy and tired and depressed as ever. And the little old hypertensive lady complained that I had only added post-operative "nerve pain" to her previous symptoms. One of the epileptic patients settled our relations and his future permanently by having himself taken from a nearby police station back to the institution where he had been.

Yet, in spite of this initial disaster, all of the other four have been for several years free from their earlier "tragic" condition (tragic no longer), or at least able to control those symptoms at will.

How was this accomplished?

Before my convalescence was completed, I knew that the operation, though beneficial, had not cured me. I had to find out why.

My next experiment was to test the effect of more

extensive surgery; the operation which had been limited to the right sympathetic chain was repeated upon the left side. The answer was prompt and rudely negative; the day after the second operation I knew I was no better. But I also was happily aware that I could probably save all my future patients the suffering and expense of the usual second stage of the lumbar sympathectomy.

During the months in which I was recovering from the second operation I did some thinking. It was obvious that some of my food-allergens remained active. But it was also obvious that I could eat many other foods to which I was now no longer allergic.

I hoped the same results could be had by the other four patients.

All were willing to try.

Success was ours in all cases. Even the two epileptic girls have solved their food-allergen problems. They now enjoy a satisfactory diet.

With the pulse-test, all five of us have found that we are now able to eat many of the foods we had to avoid before the operation.

Fortunately, no exception to this experience has yet been found. Whenever a patient's list of fool-allergens is oppressive, limited sympathectomy* is suggested. The operation has always added very many foods to the list of those that can be safely eaten.

---

*The expression "limited sympathectomy" should be explained. The popular radical sympathectomy hits the patient with the force of a major heart-attack. Even its most ardent advocate admits this. But the simple operation I recommend is quite different. A neurosurgeon described it to the parents of one of my young epileptic patients as "less formidable than tonsil removal." A "limited sympathectomy" means to remove two (sometimes only one) lumbar ganglia on one side only. The operation allows you to sit up on the third day, to walk on the fourth, and to leave the hospital (with wound healed and stitches removed) on the fifth.

# (16)

# Pulse-Dietary
# and the Doctors

Does the pulse-dietary technique fit into the present day medical practice of the general practitioner?

The consensus of those of my acquaintance who have tried it is that as things are now, it does not. There are several understandable reasons for this conclusion:

1. Few medical practitioners can spare the time to acquire the considerable experience that is necessary to enable them to interpret the pulse-dietary record.

2. After the first 3-hour educational consultation, the procedure is conducted in daily or more frequent consultations by telephone, which can be properly carried on only by the physician or a trained assistant that few afford. This requirement tends to keep the physician in the vicinity of his telephone and interferes, sometimes seriously, with his office practice. The more the physician extends the practice of pulse-dietary disease prevention, the less time he has for the orthodox practice of symptomatic treatment. He is forced to become a specialist.

3. The people for their part cannot be easily persuaded

to abandon their habit of demanding symptomatic relief of their aliments—with a pill, a "shot" or the knife.

Some would rather be ill than give up a favorite food, cigarette, or perfume; and some refuse the tests, preferring not even to know their food-poisons.

In short, because your doctor has been trained and conditioned to treat your symptoms rather than to look for the real cause of your illness, he will have a natural and understandable resistance to embracing this new and radically different approach.

There must be medical men willing to pioneer in this field and they must be willing to do it soon. Therein lies the hope.

If you have read this far, you no doubt have adequate intelligence for a trial of the method on yourself.

But what will your family doctor say? What will his reaction be?

He will rightly disapprove it if he thinks it means that the sick person is to diagnose his illness without any medical counsel. Such a man is the well-known patient who "has a fool for a doctor," and he isn't the man to whom the idea is offered.

The man or woman we have in mind *has* consulted not only his family physician, but various specialists near and far. He has learned, sometimes at huge expense, that his chronic cough is *not* tubercular; that his recurring migraine headaches are *not* caused by a tumor of his brain; that the repeated occurrence of complete loss of his voice is not due to a growth; that his indigestion, his hives, his constipation and his hemorrhoids are not serious conditions.

His doctors often begrudge the precious time this man demands from them after they have exhausted the list of pills and palliatives without relieving him. Some even tell him bluntly but honestly, "Don't come back, I can't help you."

It is this man who has a new fighting chance if he turns to the pulse-dietary method of finding the cause of his illness. He needs intelligence and a bull-dog determination to pursue his special problem to a conclusion.

He has the assurance that "there is nothing immediately serious the matter with him," and he does not need to be told that they systematic search for and avoidance of the foods which affect his pulse and make him ill is not likely to harm him.

After he has stabilized his pulse by avoidance of his food-allergens, there is time to take his list of "safe" foods to his physician for advice regarding the iron-calcium and vitamin-content and nutritive balance of his diet.

He will not be censured for self-medication since the pulse-dietary course does not represent a "treatment" at all, but a fact-finding investigation of the individual's allergic sensitivities.

The findings do often indicate measures which may be considered as treatment. For example, if the patient is found to be allergic to many foods, the conservative sympathectomy must be considered.

Some day, inevitably, the medical practitioner will come to view the pulse-dietary survey as a means of lightening the sometimes crushing burden of his practice. But the day of his deliverance will have to be postponed until that procedure has become available to his patients through the establishment of diagnostic centers under private and governmental management.

The physician has long been accustomed to the use of such technical service, which already includes X-ray (diagnostic and therapeutic), chemical and other examinations of blood, spinal fluid, stomach-contents, sputum, urine; cutaneous and other special tests too numerous to mention.

The mere equipment needed for all such technical services would dwarf the doctor's consultation rooms, and would require a sizeable staff of technicians to use it and keep it in order. The medical practitioner can no more supply his technical medical service then he can make his own penicillin.

After the pulse-survey has been completed and you, the patient, are quite well, you will report to your family physician and, if you are wise, you will heed the advice of the diagnosticians at the center to consult your doctor at regular intervals.

This will assure you of your continued freedom from any food-allergic manifestation, especially a tendency toward high blood-pressure, which may be a danger signal that you have become careless, or that a minor allergen such as house-dust may be emerging, and must be avoided.

You will have found the way to good health, and you will have found it with your own fingertips!

# Footnote:
# On Professional Acceptance

The original purpose of this book was to report to non-medical readers a new, and rather revolutionary concept of disease. It is a concept which has been slowly developing through the years, and which still lacks recognition by the controlling medical authorities.

Many of the details are matters of common knowledge and of general acceptance as allergic phenomena; but there are a number of reputedly "incurable" ailments whose allergic nature, as *suggested* in this book, will not be accepted by at least some medical specialists on the *preliminary evidence* presented here.

A highly respected medical scientist advised me that these two groups of disease be physically separated in this book, this in effect emphasizing the resistance of organized medicine to the proposed radical extension of the allergy concept.

This suggestion, I believe, overlooks the fact that "medical authority" rejects out of hand the very basic proposition that the pulse record can be used as a dependable indicator of your state of health, and as a means of identifying the specific causes of ill health.

Some medical "authorities" in institutions have refused to permit a controlled, harmless demonstration of the main principles of idioblaptic disease in patients under their control; although individual physicians have successfully applied those principles in themselves and in some of their more cooperative patients.

There seems to be no reasonable compromise of the medical principle that after a group of common ailments like headache, indigestion, constipation, eczema, abnormal tiredness and hives have been proved to be manifestations of a constitutional, hereditary allergy to foods and other substances which affect the pulse-rate; then any other chronic ailment (even if it is rated as incurable) must reasonably be suspected of the same allergic nature if in a single case it disappears after avoidance of all substances that affect the pulse-rate.

And if properly controlled future exposures to the pulse-accelerating substances cause a recurrence of the "incurable" ailment, such an observation constitutes *proof* of the allergic nature of that ailment *in that case*. In such an event, it would be, in the words of Professor Hill, "sheer madness" not to apply the pulse-method to other victims of the ailment.

The very real and discouraging problem of the resistance of medical authority to the extension of this concept of allergy is illustrated in the instance of that most common malady, headache. As long ago as 1927, the eminent allergist Warren T. Vaughan reported his original investigation of migraine headache in which he brought convincing evidence of its allergic nature.

In 1944, another distinguished allergist Herbert J. Rinkel, in a review of the literature on migraine since Vaughan's report, found that 87 percent of the papers either actively supported the allergic concept or gave approval of its possible relationship. Yet formal reviews concerning headaches have been published in recent months that have not even mentioned the possibility of an allergic nature.

Such a review was printed in an outstanding medical journal, which later rejected my own report of 53 consecutive cases of headache of all degrees having been relieved by simple avoidance of pulse-speeding foods and tobacco. The reason given for the rejection was that the results had been obtained with a method which had not been generally approved.

The censorship exercised by the higher medical authority is inevitably extended to the standard newspapers through their science editors.

The report by Dr. Milo G. Meyer of Michigan City, Indiana, Dr. Alan Johnston of Plainfield, Indiana, and me concerning the prompt arrest of multiple sclerosis in 14 of our 15 cases with antiallergic treatment, and the recurrence of symptoms in some cases on reexposure to the identified allergens, was about to be published in the *Psychiatric Quarterly* a few years ago. But an official of the society which collects funds for research in multiple sclerosis circularized its medical board, warning them that in the *opinion* of a younger member, the pulse-dietary procedure used by us "lacked merit."

It seems probable that science editors who inquired about the report at the office of that society received the same authoritatively unfavorable advice. In any case, no victim of that hopeless affliction has been referred to me by any member of that society for the complete harmless pulse-tests.

History teaches that a revolutionary idea is apt to find its most difficult resistance in a static ignorance ensconced in the seats of *power*. And it is there that out-moded opinions and practices with majority support are conscientiously maintained till nature vacates the seats and progress resumes its march.

It seems impossible to cover up the situation that has just been outlined; and it is the writer's hope and expectation that the discussion of it may not add resentment to the rather general skepticism toward the novel idea of disease-prevention.

Those physicians of all ages who are themselves subjects of serious chronic ailments may be stimulated by this book to apply the diagnostic method to themselves. The more open minded and determined among these will succeed, and in so doing will become the convinced leaders of the new "preventive medicine."

It is hoped too that this book may serve as an instruction manual which will greatly lighten the physician's labor with his patients.

# MIND MEETS BODY...
# HEALTH MEETS HAPPINESS...
# SPIRIT MEETS SERENITY...

In his writings, spiritual advisor Edgar Cayce counseled thousands with his extraordinary, yet practical guidance to the mind/body/spirit connection. Now, the Edgar Cayce series, based on actual readings by the renowned psychic, can provide you with insights in the search for understanding and meaning in life.

**KEYS TO HEALTH**: The Promise and Challenge of Holism
Eric A. Mein, M.D.
_____ 95616-9 $4.99 U.S./$5.99 CAN.

**REINCARNATION**: Claiming Your Past, Creating Your Future
Lynn Elwell Sparrow
_____ 95754-8 $4.99 U.S./$5.99 CAN.

**DREAMS**: Tonight's Answers for Tomorrow's Questions
Mark Thurston, Ph.D.
_____ 95771-8 $5.50 U.S./$6.50 CAN.

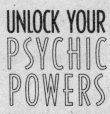

We've all been there—angry at ourselves for overeating, for our lack of willpower, for failing at yet another diet that was supposed to be the last one. But the problem is not you, it's that dieting, with its emphasis on rules and regulations, has stopped you from listening to your body. Now you can rediscover the pleasures of eating and rebuild your body image.

# INTUITIVE EATING

## EVELYN TRIBOLE, M.S., R.D.
## AND ELYSE RESCH, M.S., R.D.